Pectus Excavatum and Poland Syndrome Surgery

Jean-Pierre Chavoin

Editor

Pectus Excavatum and Poland Syndrome Surgery

Custom-Made Silicone Implants by
Computer Aided Design

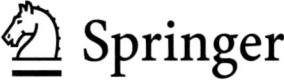 Springer

Editor
Jean-Pierre Chavoin
Plastic Surgery Department
Rangueil Hospital, Toulouse University Hospital
Toulouse
France

ISBN 978-3-030-05107-5   ISBN 978-3-030-05108-2   (eBook)
https://doi.org/10.1007/978-3-030-05108-2

Library of Congress Control Number: 2019930167

This Springer imprint is published by the registered company Springer Nature Switzerland AG
The registered company address is: Gewerbestrasse 11, 6330 Cham, Switzerland

Preface

Congenital chest abnormalities such as pectus excavatum and Poland syndrome are well known to be mostly a real psychological and social problem because of this morphological difference and asymmetries.

Research on the genetic background and a probable vascular embryologic origin of these outbreaks is very interesting (Chaput); mostly, these can be associated with each other or with other conditions like tuberous breasts in women. The fibrous network could be induced by a lack of vascularization so that the normal growth of cartilage, muscles, and breasts is stopped or slowed down.

Pectus excavatum is by far the most common with at least 1/1000 patients, but it is difficult to obtain statistics on this malformation which is not often seen at birth as in the case of Poland (1/30,000). In addition, many patients have mild deformity and asymmetry that are not obvious for physicians, as there are no functional disorders and surgical solutions are too invasive. The respiratory (Daussy) and cardiac (Shah) functions seem to be, in most cases, compatible with a normal life: the benefit/risk balance clearly supports plastic surgeries because they offer good aesthetic results, postoperative pain is very low, and significant complications are extremely rare.

Many Thoracic surgeons have given their experience in this book: Marcel Dahan since 25 years in Toulouse and more recently Ian Hunt and Samir Shah in London, Elisabeth Barthe Le Pimpec in Paris; thanks for their essential contribution, help and confidence.

Custom-made implants offer a very good solution since they are made with a soft silicone elastomer and put under the pectoralis muscle and rectus sheath for pectus, under the skin, or under the breast for Poland after a perfectly precise computer-aided design (CAD) based on a CT scan (Chavoin, Moreno).

These procedures are done at the same time, in less than 1 h, and the implants will be retained throughout the lifetime, without infections, rupture, or capsular retraction. These are much less invasive than orthopedic procedures, which are also described in this book by a thoracic surgeon (Hunt) who proposes three types of surgery for a complete information of the patients according to their real problem.

Indeed literature is very rich to describe problems or complications which can occur with these brilliant but invasive procedures. Furthermore, many pediatric and thoracic surgeons ask to be trained or informed about this CAD custom-made implant's technique, firstly to improve some poor results due to recurrences, persistent asymmetry, or others and then for primary corrections when the indication is not clearly functional.

The CAD custom-made implant procedure is now achieved and used throughout the world.

Our personal experience of 25 years, 600 pectus, and 140 Poland wouldn't have existed without the patients' formal consent and satisfaction in terms of comfort and results.

We hope that this book will convince other surgeons to enhance their results and decrease their stress, risks for their patients, and possible legal implications.

Toulouse, France   Jean-Pierre Chavoin

Foreword

The problem of major deformities of the chest wall has been controversial for several decades between the different specialties that support it: thus, thoracic surgeons favor radical methods after growth (Ravitch), infant surgeons propose orthopedic methods (corset) or mini-invasives (Nuss) willingly before puberty, and finally plastic surgeons who use prostheses try to apply it to the thorax. The cardiorespiratory effect is the choice argument of the "maximalists"; the purely aesthetic demand, that of the minimalists; and the psychological impact, of pediatricians. The truth is certainly a compromise that will appear when we answer the following three questions fairly: At what age to intervene—before or after growth? Surgical or medical methods? Modeling surgery or simple prosthesis? From an ethical point of view, we find it illegitimate to propose an intervention with serious consequences to an individual whose only demand remains cosmetic. Also, with the experience of our fellow plastic surgeons described in this book, in the pectus excavatum without proven cardiorespiratory consequences, we favor the installation of premolded prostheses, a technique characterized by its simplicity, safety, and reversibility: simple because a short incision and a day of hospitalization are enough, safe because it respects and, what is more, protects even the chest wall, and reversible because change and ablation are easy to perform. Unlike other "invasive" techniques, it does not indicate any "physical" occupation and does not require subsequent thoracic surgery. Thus, the experience of our colleagues in biocompatible materials and 3D reconstruction has allowed us for over 25 years to adopt their techniques and perform interventions whose immediate aesthetic result is striking. Reading this book by Professor Chavoin, you will certainly find the quest of a practitioner open to other specialties and looking for a compromise between an aesthetic result in line with the patient's request and a surgical gesture really "mini-invasive."

Toulouse, France   Marcel Dahan
Paris, France   Françoise Le Pimpec Barthes

Contents

1 **Thoracic Malformations: Etiopathogeny, Genetic,
and Associated Syndromes**.   1
Benoit Chaput, Alexane Laguerre, and Jean-Pierre Chavoin

2 **Computer-Aided Design: Prototyping and Manufacturing
(Pectus Excavatum and Poland Syndrome)**   13
Benjamin Moreno, Pierre Leyx, and Jean-Pierre Chavoin

3 **Pectus Excavatum Remodelling by CAD Custom-Made
Silicone Implant: Experience of 600 Cases**.   35
Jean-Pierre Chavoin, Marcel Dahan, Benjamin Moreno,
Jean-Louis Grolleau, and Benoit Chaput

4 **Poland Syndrome Remodeling by CAD Silicone
Custom-Made Implants**   57
Jean-Pierre Chavoin, Mohcine Taizou, Benjamin Moreno,
Jean-Louis Grolleau, and Benoit Chaput

5 **Breasts and Pectus Excavatum**   71
Jean-Pierre Chavoin, Mary Morgan, Richard Vaucher,
Benjamin Moreno, Benoit Chaput, and Jean-Louis Grolleau

6 **Filling Method with Fat Graft Technique in Pectus
Excavatum and Poland Syndrome**   89
Christian Herlin

7 **Thoracic Surgical Correction of Pectus Excavatum:
Minimal and Open Approaches**.   99
Ian Hunt and Stephanie Fraser

8 **Pectus Excavatum: Functional Respiratory Impact,
Quality of Life, and Preoperative Assessment** 115
Louis Daussy, Elise Noel-Savina, Alain Didier, and Daniel Riviere

9   The Cardiorespiratory Implications of Pectus Excavatum. 125
      Samir S. Shah and Pankaj Kumar Mishra

**10   Complications and Hazards with Pectus Excavatum Surgeries:
      Secondary Surgical Procedures with Implants** 133
      Françoise Le Pimpec Barthes, Ian Hunt, Samir S. Shah,
      Antonio Messineo, Louis Daussy, Aymeric André, Marcel Dahan,
      and Jean-Pierre Chavoin

Thoracic Malformations: Etiopathogeny, Genetic, and Associated Syndromes

Benoit Chaput, Alexane Laguerre,
and Jean-Pierre Chavoin

1.1 Introduction

Chest malformations are an issue that it is common to be confronted with in plastic and reconstructive surgery. The panel of these malformations is relatively large, and it happens that several thoracic malformations are associated with each other. Also, some chest deformities will be associated with limb deformities, face or deeper tissue and visceral anomalies, and thus integrate into larger syndromes. It is essential to always have in mind when dealing with these patients, the screening and management of these associated malformations.

Congenital chest wall deformities can be classified into rare entities such as the cleft sternum, pentalogy of Cantrell, asphyxiating thoracic dystrophy (Jeune syndrome), Poland syndrome, and spondylothoracic dysplasia (Jarcho–Levin syndrome), representing 3–4% of all cases, and frequent entities PE and pectus carinatum representing 95–97% [1].

The pathogenesis of chest deformities is often misidentified or hypothetical because it differs according to the type of malformation. In fact, our true knowledge of pathogenesis is often based on observation or deductions from historical description or notions. Poland syndrome and pectus excavatum (PE) and the syndromes sometimes associated are varied.

B. Chaput · A. Laguerre · J.-P. Chavoin (✉)
Plastic Surgery Department, Rangueil Hospital, Toulouse University Hospital, Toulouse, France
e-mail: chaput.b@chu-toulouse.fr; alex.laguerre@laposte.net; jean-pierre.chavoin@orange.fr

© Springer Nature Switzerland AG 2019   1
J.-P. Chavoin (ed.), *Pectus Excavatum and Poland Syndrome Surgery*,
https://doi.org/10.1007/978-3-030-05108-2_1

In this chapter, we will discuss the different embryological or genetic etiologies of PE and Poland syndrome, and the different associations that can be found more or less frequently.

1.2   Pectus Excavatum or Funnel Chest

PE is the most common congenital chest malformation. The etiology of PE remains relatively poorly explained, however proposed theories for its development include abnormal intrauterine pressure, rickets, pulmonary restriction, and abnormalities of the diaphragm that result in posterior traction on the sternum [2–6]. A genetic or embryological etiology has already been mentioned and in some cases there is a family history. We find associated with PE, thoracic or spinal malformations such as Poland syndrome (Fig. 1.1) or idiopathic scoliosis, breast malformations such as tuberous breasts or more rarely, polymalformative syndromes such as Noonan syndrome, Marfan or Turner (Fig. 1.2).

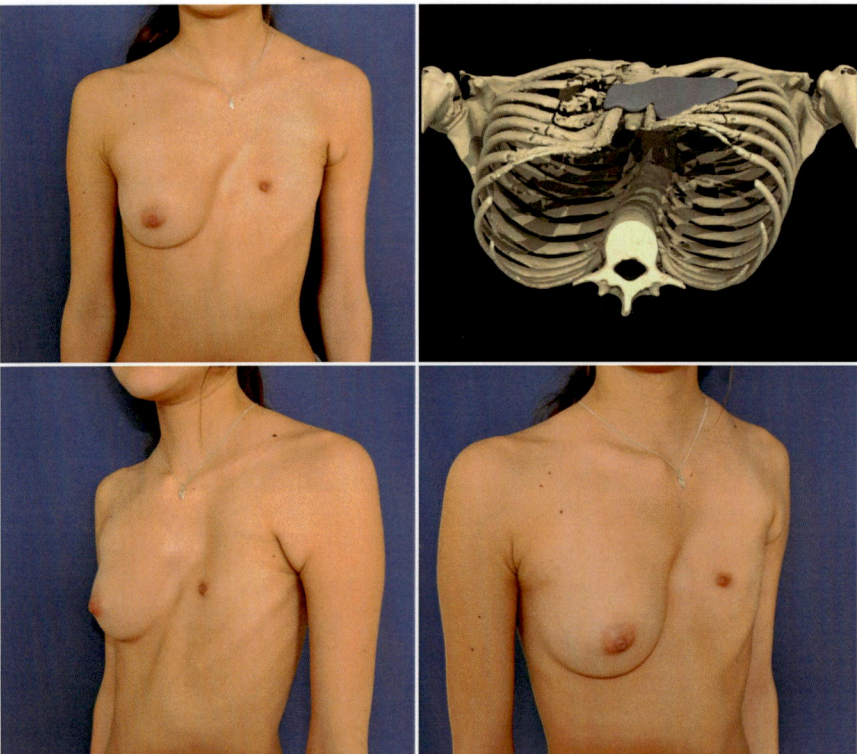

Fig. 1.1 Pectus excavatum associated with a Poland syndrome on the left side in a 19-year-old woman

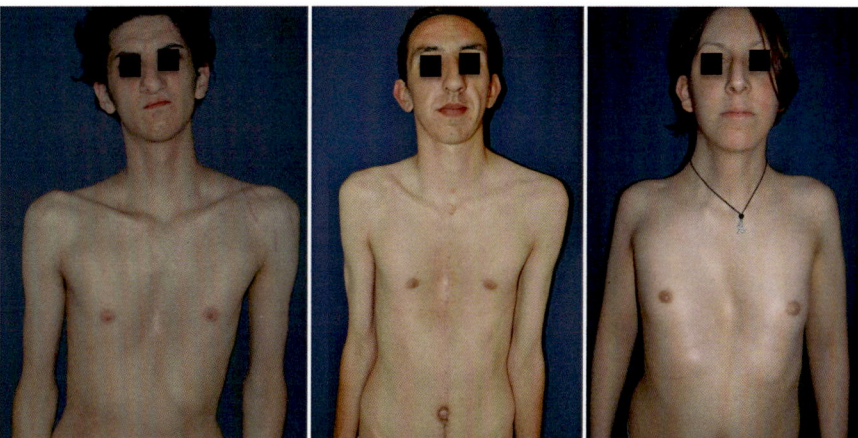

Fig. 1.2 Pectus excavatum in Marfan syndrome (*Left and middle*). Pectus excavatum in a Turner syndrome; note the pterygium colli before surgical correction

Embryology's knowledge of the chest wall is essential for understanding PE. Embryologic development of the ribs begins during the fifth week, with the outgrowth of the distal tips of the vertebrae's costal processes on thorax. In the mid of the sixth week, the first seven ribs (true ribs) have connected ventrally with the sternum via costal cartilages. The lower five ribs do not articulate directly with the sternum and are called the false ribs [7]. Late in the sixth week, the ribs separate from the vertebrae through the formation of the costovertebral joints. The ribs begin as cartilaginous precursors that later ossify by endochondral ossification. In the sixth week, primary ossification centers form near the angle of each rib. Secondary ossification develops in the tubercles and heads of the ribs during adolescence. At the end of the sixth week, there is formation of paired mesenchymal condensations termed sternal bars within the ventrolateral body wall. In the seventh week, the most cranial ribs fuse with these sternal bars. The bars meet at the midline and fusion begins with the most cranial end and proceeds towards the caudal end, concluding with the formation of the xiphoid process in the ninth week. Similar to the ribs, the sternal bones originate as cartilaginous precursors. Ossification of the sternal bones also occurs in a cranio-caudal direction [7]. The mesosternum begins as four inter-segmental sternabrae and fuses during puberty. Costal cartilages are persistent, unossified, anterior components of the precursors from which the ribs develop. From the first to the seventh rib, the cartilages consecutively increase in length, then decrease from the seventh to the 12th [8]. The main source of blood to the sternum originates from the internal thoracic artery.

There exist several hypotheses regarding PE pathogenesis. Bauhinus gave the first pathophysiological hypothesis mentioning a hypertension of the diaphragm during embryonic development [9]. Until beginning of the twentieth century, one leading opinion on pathogenesis was intrauterine pressure on the sternum through an abnormal position of the embryo [10, 11]. Further hypotheses highlighted other diseases such as syphilis or rickets as the reason for PE. In contrast, Brown published in 1939 his observations of a thickened ligamentum substernale, which should lead to a retraction of the sternum [12]. A further hypothesis favored an imbalance between the anterior and posterior musculature of the muscle fibers of the anterior part of the diaphragm with a movement of the xiphoid and sternum backwards. Today's leading hypotheses focused on two main etiologies, an overgrowth of the sternocostal cartilage or a defective metabolism in the sternocostal cartilage, resulting in a biomechanical weakness [13].

1.2.1 Developmental Theory

Sweet hypothesized that the cause of PE is overgrowth of the costal cartilage. This hypothesis was widely accepted as the cause of PE. However, no evidence demonstrating this hypothesis has been reported [13]. Nakaoka et al. wanted to check the theory of overgrowth of the costal cartilage. According to this hypothesis, the length of costal cartilages must be longer in the side of deep depression in asymmetric patients. To challenge this analysis, they measured the lengths of ribs and costal cartilages and investigated lateral differences in two studies [14, 15]. Twenty-four adolescent and adult patients with asymmetric PE were evaluated. They investigated the length of the fifth and sixth costal cartilages and ribs in PE patients from reconstructed images of three-dimensional computed tomography. To examine the relative costal cartilage length, they calculated the C/R ratio, defined as the quotient of the costal cartilage length divided by the adjacent rib length and compared it between PE patients and healthy controls [15]. In PE patients, the C/R ratios were not larger than in healthy controls at any level. At the left sixth, the C/R ratio was significantly smaller in patients than in the healthy control group. The results revealed that, in PE patients, relative costal cartilage lengths were not longer than in healthy controls. They conclude that the overgrowth of costal cartilage is not the etiology of PE.

Thus, this first hypothesis seems still unverified and additional investigations are essential.

1.2.2 Metabolic Theory

A systematic analysis of the histological changes in the sternocostal cartilage of PE patients revealed a premature aging of the cartilage [16]. Regarding the cause for an inadequate degradation, an ultrastructural and biochemical study demonstrated abnormalities in the content of trace elements in the costal cartilage from PE patients, namely decreased levels of zinc and increased levels of magnesium and calcium [17], which demonstrated that the lack of zinc in the diet results in a lower metabolic activity of chondrocytes. Feng et al. were able to demonstrate the deficit of the biomechanical qualities in the cartilage from PE patients [18]. These findings give interesting insights in the correlation of metabolic lesions and mechanical properties of the cartilage in PE.

1.2.3 Genetic Theory

The hereditary nature of the PE has often been mentioned. In 1934, a student in a genetics class at Ohio State University came forward with an atypic looking chest and after investigation it was found that eight members of his family all had similar conditions [19]. Upon naming the deformity koilosternia (PE), Snyder and Curtis concluded that this deformity followed an autosomal dominant pattern of inheritance [19]. Stoddard reported genetic linkage in a family with 49 cases of PE spanning over four generations. This author also hypothesized autosomal dominant transmission. Despite Stoddard's report, records of familial nonsyndromic PE are limited [20] and the presence of mild Marfan syndrome or any other monogenic syndrome cannot be ruled out [21]. Approximately 40% of patients with PE deformities have family members who also have similar defects [22].

Creswick et al. in 2006 have studied 34 families with more than one affected individual by PE [5]. A total of 14 families suggested autosomal dominant inheritance, four families suggested autosomal recessive inheritance, six families suggested X-linked recessive inheritance, and ten families had complex inheritance patterns. Creswick et al. concluded that PE is an inherited disorder, possibly of connective tissue genes defects, such as fibrillin, collagen, and transforming growth factor β. And although some families demonstrate apparent Mendelian inheritance, most of them appear to be multifactorial with unknown environmental factors [5]. In 2009, Gurnett et al. performed a genetic linkage analysis in a single large family in which adolescent idiopathic scoliosis (AIS) and PE segregate as an autosomal dominant condition. They highlighted a novel locus for AIS and PE on chromosome 18q12.1-q12.2 [23].

Wu et al. have analyzed a four-generation Chinese family with PE that showed dominant inheritance. Through whole-exome sequencing of this family with congenital PE, they identified mutations in the sulfotransferase gene *GAL3ST4* (galactose-3-*O*-sulfotransferase 4) [24]. Previous studies highlighted that sulfation of the proteoglycans is essential for the normal development of cartilages and bones [25]. Wu et al. consider that this is the first gene linked to the pathogenesis of PE.

More recently, Karner CM et al. found that loss of *GPR126* upregulated the expression of *GAL3ST4* (implicated in human PE) [26]. G protein-coupled receptor 126 also known as VIGR and DREG is a protein encoded by the *ADGRG6* gene. They demonstrate that *GPR126*, a gene implicated in human AIS, acts in axial cartilage to regulate normal spine and sternum development in mouse [27]. Loss of *GPR126* in cartilage tissues results in defects of the axial column and increased apoptosis in *GPR126* suggests a common pathophysiology for AIS and PE. They highlighted *GPR126* as a genetic cause for the pathogenesis of adolescent idiopathic scoliosis and PE in a mouse model [26].

Correlations of adolescent idiopathic scoliosis and PE have been studied by Hong et al. on 248 patients with PE [28]. Overall, 56 of the 248 study patients had scoliosis (Cobb angle >10°), a prevalence of 22.58%. PE and AIS were found to have a high concomitant incidence. Surgeons should consider these relationships when deciding upon treatment in patients with chest and spinal deformities.

Truncal distortion with rib deformity is probably the main etiology of PE, which is reminiscent of scoliosis, which often shows vertebral rotation, rib hump, and sternal deformities [28]. The prevalence of AIS has been reported to range from 0.5 to 3% [28].

The most frequently observed monogenic syndromes associated with PE are Noonan syndrome and Marfan syndrome [21]. PE or carinatum are a hallmark of Marfan syndrome, a systemic disorder of connective tissue, which is caused by mutations in the Fibrillin 1, a gene localized on the long arm of chromosome 15. Prevalence of this autosomal dominantly inherited disorder is around 1:5–10,000. Penetrance is almost 100% with broad interfamiliar and intrafamiliar variability ranging from isolated features to severe presentation already in neonates and poor genotype–phenotype correlation. Recurrence risk for a patient's children is 50%. A clinical diagnosis of Marfan syndrome is possible, if symptoms of at least two major organ systems (ocular [myopia, lens dislocation, retinal detachment], cardiovascular [dilatation or dissection of the ascending aorta, mitral, or tricuspid valve prolapse], dural ectasia, and skeletal [dolichostenomelia, scoliosis]) or a family history or a Fibrillin 1 mutation and a minor manifestation of one of the other organ systems are present [29].

Noonan syndrome is a common autosomal dominantly inherited disorder caused by mutations in various genes in the RasMAPK (mitogen-activated protein kinase) pathway [30]. The RAS (RAt Sarcoma viral oncogene homolog) proteins and their downstream pathways are a signaling cascade important for cell proliferation, differentiation, survival, and cell death. The phenotype is characterized by normal measurements at birth but short stature in adulthood. We can see congenital heart defects (with pulmonary valve stenosis 20–30%) and/or cardiomyopathy (20–30%), broad or webbed neck, cranial pectus carinatum, and caudal pectus excavatum; cryptorchidism (60–80%), coagulation defects; and facial dysmorphisms including ptosis, wide-spaced eyes, and low-set and posteriorly rotated ears. Some of these features are because of jugular lymphatic obstructions. Aortic dilatation is more common in the presence of PE and its complications are a significant cause of morbidity and mortality in Marfan syndrome. PE is also associated with distorted right ventricular geometry and reduced ejection fraction, abnormalities readily detected and monitored by CMR [31]. Mental development is variable.

In our experience of 600 cases, we found frequent associations with breast asymmetry (32) or tuberous breasts, and less frequently abnormalities integrating into polymalformative syndromes (less than 10% of cases). Apart from polymalformative syndromes, PE etiologies are multiple and the multifactorial nature of PE is not to be ruled out. As many authors, we are convinced that PE is very rarely associated with a cardiopulmonary repercussion on which a remodeling chest surgery could have a positive effect. On the other hand, the association of PE with other syndromes must make us keep in mind that it is not always an isolated physical symptom but that it sometimes fits into a more complex syndromic entity. This is why its management must remain a case of surgeon specialized in this pathology.

1.3   Poland Syndrome

In 1841, a medical student, Sir Alfred Poland, based on an autopsy of a 27-year-old man, described a new syndrome characterized by a complete unilateral absence of the m. pectoralis major, m. serratus anterior, and m. obliquus externus abdominis with ipsilateral thoracic and upper limb defects [32].

In 1972, for David TJ in the New England Journal of Medicine, the essential features of Poland syndrome are unilateral absence of the sternocostal head of the pectoralis major muscle and ipsilateral syndactyly [33]. We currently know that the procession of malformations associated with the Poland syndrome is actually much larger, especially in the upper limb (Fig. 1.3).

In an etiopathogenic level, David TJ had evoked unsuccessful abortion for half of the 10 patients he had supported and others, deformities of prematurity or the use of medication with teratogenicity [33]. At present, different etiologic factors of the Poland syndrome are discussed: genetic, vascular disruption during embryogenesis and also teratogenic effect (e.g., cigarette smoking during pregnancy, viral infections).

1.3.1   Vascular Theory

Bavinck and Weaver suggested that Poland syndrome is a result of an interruption of the early embryonic blood supply in the subclavian arteries, the vertebral arteries, and/or their branches. They introduced the term "subclavian artery supply disruption sequence" (SASDS) [34]. This is the most advanced theory at the moment. A partial or complete interruption of blood flow in the subclavian or vertebral arteries and/or their branches during or shortly before horizons 17 and 18 would be responsible for absence of the pectoralis major, failure of degeneration of interdigital tissue, and failure of segmentation of cervical vertebrae. According to the authors,

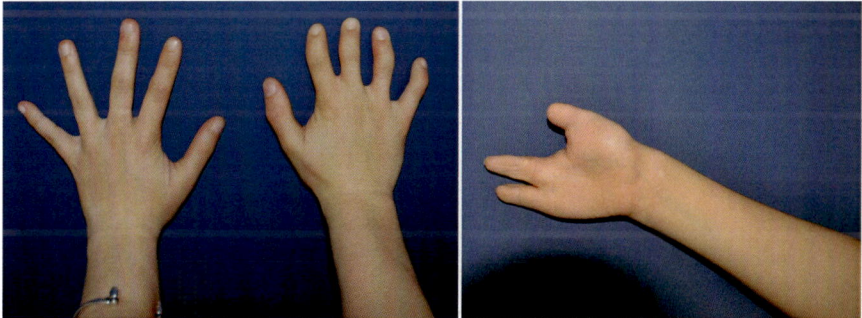

Fig. 1.3 Brachymesophalangy on the right hand; one of the most common malformations of Poland syndrome (*Left*). Complex malformation of the right hand with adactylia of the second and third digital ray and hypoplasia of the thumb (*Right*). This malformation is much less common

interruption of the internal thoracic artery leads to absence of the pectoralis major and ipsilateral breast hypoplasia. Interruption of the subclavian artery distal to the origin of the internal thoracic artery causes isolated terminal transverse limb defects. Interruption of the subclavian artery proximal to the origin of the internal thoracic artery but distal to the origin of the vertebral artery leads to the Poland anomaly. Interruption of blood flow in the subclavian artery distal to the origin of the internal thoracic artery could produce isolated defects of the arm and hand. During horizon 18, the interdigital spaces in the hand are normally formed by degeneration of inter-digital webs. Ischemia before or during this period might lead to arrest in the degen-eration of these webs and the formation of digits and the defects seen in this condition, as syndactyly and hypoplasia or absence of distal structures.

The hypothesis of subclavian artery malformation was strongly supported by Bouvet et al., who showed differences of the velocity of the systolic increase in the arterial volume between the two arms (normal arm vs. arm with congenital anom-aly) in patients with Poland syndrome [35]. Bouvet studied 8 children with the Poland anomaly using impedance plethysmography and showed marked decreases in arterial blood flow velocities in the affected sides, suggesting hypoplasia in the subclavian artery [35]. These results, which are also observed in stenotic atheroscle-rosis, support the hypothesis of hypoplasia of the ipsilateral subclavian artery as the origin of the malformation; nonetheless, a local anomaly in arterial-wall viscosity remains possible.

Possible causes for interruption or reduction of blood flow in the subclavian arter-ies and their branches are intrinsic mechanical factors such as blood vessel edema, thrombi, and emboli, which can obstruct the lumen and external pressure on the blood vessels by edema of the surrounding tissue, hemorrhage, cervical rib, aberrant muscle, amnion rupture/amniotic bands, early intrauterine compression, or a tumor [34]. Certain normal embryologic events might predispose the embryo to the devel-opment of vascular obstructions and the SASDS. Specific configurations of the embryonic blood vessels at certain times during morphogenesis may increase the chance of developing vascular occlusion. Alternatively, there may be abnormal events in the development of the blood vessels such as delayed vessel formation, structural or anatomical abnormalities of the blood vessels, disruption of newly formed vessels, and premature disappearance of transient vessels. All these events can be precipitated by environmental factors, such as infection (i.e., rubella), hyper-thermia, generalized hypoxia, drugs. Multiple mechanisms may operate to produce the subclavian artery supply disruption sequence. For instance, the development of the U-shaped configuration of the subclavian artery during horizon 18 and later might make this vessel more susceptible to compression by external mechanical fac-tors, such as the first rib, a cervical rib, or the anterior scalene muscle, or by obstruc-tion from within the vessel. Emboli and thrombi can also impede blood. Furthermore, the tortuous nature of the longitudinal anastomoses that form the vertebral arteries (horizons 16–18) may make these vessels more prone to obstruction.

Finally, vascular theory could thus explain the mammary malformations as hypoplasia or tuberous breasts that are found in some patients with Poland syn-drome (Fig. 1.4).

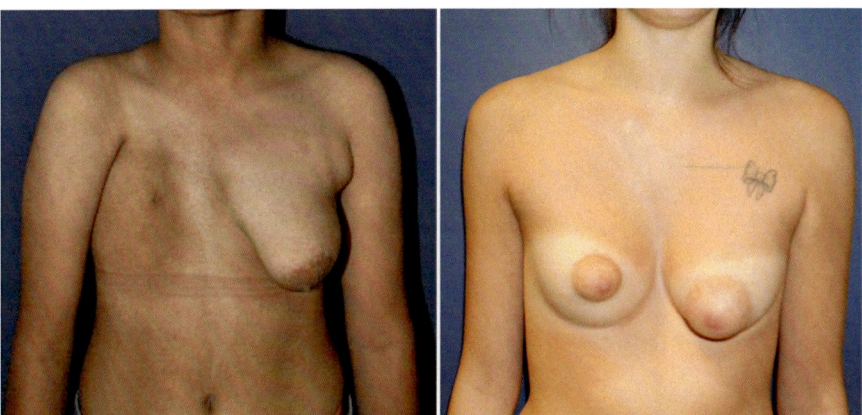

Fig. 1.4 (*Left*) Poland syndrome associated with tuberous breast type 2. (*Right*) Pectus excavatum associated with asymmetric tuberous breast (type 2 bilateral) in a 19-year-old woman

1.3.2 Embryologic Theory

Bamforth puis Sparks proposed an alternative theory [36, 37] in which it is suggested that the anomaly results from a failure of the paraxial mesenchyme to develop. Sparks described the case of a 57-year-old man that can be best explained by an isolated defect in the paraxial mesenchyme during early limb development, rather than an interruption in the blood supply to the muscle. This theory is nevertheless not very well supported by other authors.

1.3.3 Genetic Theory

The genetic etiology seems much less convincing than for the PE. Besides the literature, it does not actually exist gene identified in the development of this syndrome at present except in a case report of Vaccari et al. [38]. The authors describe a couple of monozygotic (MZ) twin girls, both presenting with Poland syndrome. The twins carry a de novo heterozygous *126KBP* deletion at chromosome 11q12.3 involving five genes, four of which, namely *HRASLS5*, *RARRES3*, *HRASLS2*, and *PLA2G16*, encoding proteins that regulate cellular growth, differentiation, and apoptosis, mainly through Ras-mediated signaling pathways. Phenotype concordance between the monozygotic twin probands provides evidence supporting the genetic control of Poland syndrome. As genes controlling cell growth and differentiation may be related to morphological defects originating during development, Vaccari et al. postulate that the observed chromosome deletion could be causative of the phenotype observed in the twin girls and the deleted genes could play a role in Poland syndrome development.

Nonetheless, most of the described cases are sporadic, rare familial incidence of Poland syndrome has been reported (Fig. 1.5). For example, Sierra Santos and González Rodríguez describe the occurrence of Poland syndrome in two cousins but

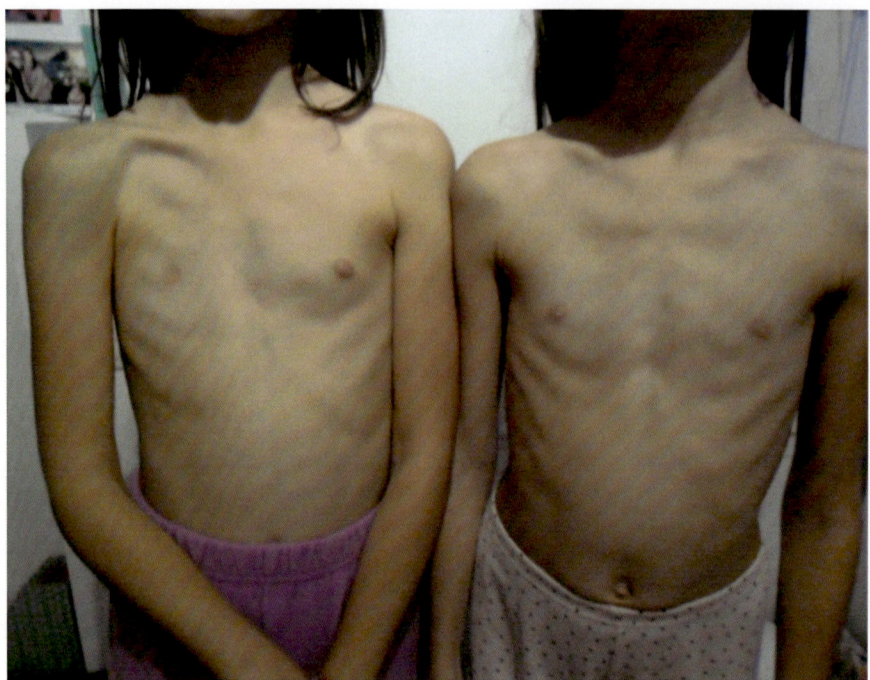

Fig. 1.5 True twin but Poland syndrome is present only in one of them

these cases are exceptional [39]. Genetic theories and hereditary transmissions therefore seem to us totally discarded.

Other hypotheses for possible development of Poland syndrome are mechanical insults (trauma of mother's abdomen, amniotic bands or pressure on umbilical cord), infections, or atrophy of the motor neurons of anterior horns of the spinal cord [40, 41]. However, these hypotheses seem to be less presumable.

1.4   Conclusion

Chest wall defects can be an isolated malformation or dysmorphic feature or only one symptom of a genetic syndrome. On the etiopathogenic level, the EP seems rather multifactorial but with a certain genetic component, whereas for the Poland syndrome, the initial vascular theory remains the most probable. But the *primum movens* of the vascular theory is totally ignored. Every patient with a chest wall deformity should be carefully evaluated for additional symptoms not only of the skeleton but also of other organ systems. Ultimately, could the syndromic association be a negative factor for surgical management? PE and Poland syndrome can therefore be the "point of call" for larger malformation syndrome and if any genetic syndrome is suspected, the patient should be referred for genetic counseling to confirm the syndromic diagnosis and to discuss karyotyping or possible molecular investigation, so as to guide our management.

References

1. Brochhausen C, et al. Pectus excavatum: history, hypotheses and treatment options. Interact Cardiovasc Thorac Surg. 2012;14(6):801–6.
2. Brown AL, Cook O. Funnel chest (pectus excavatum) in infancy and adult life. Calif Med. 1951;74(3):174–8.
3. Chin EF. Surgery of funnel chest and congenital sternal prominence. Br J Surg. 1957;44(186):360–76.
4. Lester CW. The surgical treatment of funnel chest. Ann Surg. 1946;123(6):1003–22.
5. Creswick HA, et al. Family study of the inheritance of pectus excavatum. J Pediatr Surg. 2006;41(10):1699–703.
6. Ravitch MM. The operative treatment of pectus excavatum. Ann Surg. Apr. 1949;129(4):429–44.
7. Schoenwolf GC, Bleyl SB, Brauer PR, Francis-West PH. Larsen's human embryology. 4th ed. Philadelphia: Churchill Livingstone; 2009. p. 227–8.
8. Standring S. Chest wall and breast. In: Gray's anatomy. 40th ed. New York: Churchill Livingstone; 2008. p. 915–38.
9. Bauhinus J. Observatio. In: *Ioannis Schenckii a Grafenberg*, ed. Johannes Observatorium medicarum, rararum, novarum, admirabilium, et montrosarum, liber secundus. Frankfurt: De partibus vitalibus, thorace contentis; 1609. p. 322.
10. Williams C. Congenital malformation of the thorax great depression of the sternum. Trans Path Soc. 1872;24:50.
11. Langer E. Zuckerkandel: Untersuchungen über den mißbildeten Brustkorb des. Herrn JW Wiener med Zeit. 1880;49:515.
12. Brown A. Pectus excavatum (funnel chest). J Thorac Surg. 1939;(9):164–84.
13. Sweet RH. Pectus excavatum: report of two cases successfully operated upon. Ann Surg. 1944;119(6):922–34.
14. Nakaoka T, Uemura S, Yano T, Nakagawa Y, Tanimoto T, Suehiro S. Does overgrowth of costal cartilage cause pectus excavatum? A study on the lengths of ribs and costal cartilages in asymmetric patients. J Pediatr Surg. 2009;44(7):1333–6.
15. Nakaoka T, Uemura S, Yoshida T, Tanimoto T, Miyake H. Overgrowth of costal cartilage is not the etiology of pectus excavatum. J Pediatr Surg. 2010;45(10):2015–8.
16. Geisbe H, Buddecke E, Flach A, Müller G, Stein U. [88. Biochemical, morphological and physical as well as animal experimental studies on the pathogenesis of funnel chest]. Langenbecks Arch Chir. 1967;319:536–41.
17. Rupprecht H, Hümmer HP, Stöss H, Waldherr T. [Pathogenesis of chest wall abnormalities–electron microscopy studies and trace element analysis of rib cartilage]. Z Kinderchir. 1987;42(4):228–9.
18. Feng J, et al. The biomechanical, morphologic, and histochemical properties of the costal cartilages in children with pectus excavatum. J Pediatr Surg. 2001;36(12):1770–6.
19. Snyder LH, Curtis GM. An inherited 'hollow CHEST. J Hered. 1934;25(11):445–7.
20. Stoddard SE. The inheritance of 'hollow CHEST'. J Hered. 1939;30(4):139–41.
21. Kotzot D, Schwabegger AH. Etiology of chest wall deformities–a genetic review for the treating physician. J Pediatr Surg. 2009;44(10):2004–11.
22. Dean C, Etienne D, Hindson D, Matusz P, Tubbs RS, Loukas M. Pectus excavatum (funnel chest): a historical and current prospective. Surg Radiol Anat. 2012;34(7):573–9.
23. Gurnett CA, et al. Genetic linkage localizes an adolescent idiopathic scoliosis and pectus excavatum gene to chromosome 18 q. Spine (Phila Pa 1976). 2009;34(2):E94–100.
24. Wu S, et al. Evidence for GAL3ST4 mutation as the potential cause of pectus excavatum. Cell Res. 2012;22(12):1712–5.
25. Honke K, Taniguchi N. Sulfotransferases and sulfated oligosaccharides. Med Res Rev. 2002;22(6):637–54.
26. Karner CM, Long F, Solnica-Krezel L, Monk KR, Gray RS. Gpr126/Adgrg6 deletion in cartilage models idiopathic scoliosis and pectus excavatum in mice. Hum Mol Genet. 2015;24(15):4365–73.

27. Kou I, et al. Genetic variants in GPR126 are associated with adolescent idiopathic scoliosis. Nat Genet. 2013;45(6):676–9.
28. Hong J-Y, Suh S-W, Park H-J, Kim Y-H, Park J-H, Park S-Y. Correlations of adolescent idiopathic scoliosis and pectus excavatum. J Pediatr Orthop. 2011;31(8):870–4.
29. De Paepe A, Devereux RB, Dietz HC, Hennekam RC, Pyeritz RE. Revised diagnostic criteria for the Marfan syndrome. Am J Med Genet. 1996;62(4):417–26.
30. Allanson JE. Noonan syndrome. Am J Med Genet C Semin Med Genet. 2007;145C(3):274–9.
31. Jabbour A, Zaman S, Ismail T, Prasad S, Mohiaddin R. Profound pectus excavatum in Marfan's syndrome. Lancet (London, England). 2012;379(9815):557.
32. Poland A. Deficiency of the pectoral muscles. Guys Hosp Rep. 1841;6:191–3.
33. David TJ. Nature and etiology of the Poland anomaly. N Engl J Med. 1972;287(10):487–9.
34. Bavinck JN, Weaver DD. Subclavian artery supply disruption sequence: hypothesis of a vascular etiology for Poland, Klippel-Feil, and Möbius anomalies. Am J Med Genet. 1986;23(4):903–18.
35. Bouvet JP, Leveque D, Bernetieres F, Gros JJ. Vascular origin of Poland syndrome? A comparative rheographic study of the vascularisation of the arms in eight patients. Eur J Pediatr. 1978;128(1):17–26.
36. Bamforth JS, Fabian C, Machin G, Honore L. Poland anomaly with a limb body wall disruption defect: case report and review. Am J Med Genet. 1992;43(5):780–4.
37. Sparks DS, Adams BM, Wagels M. Poland's syndrome: an alternative to the 'vascular hypothesis'. Surg Radiol Anat. 2015;37(6):701–2.
38. Vaccari CM, et al. De novo deletion of chromosome 11q12.3 in monozygotic twins affected by Poland syndrome. BMC Med Genet. 2014;15(1):63.
39. Sierra Santos L, González Rodríguez MP. [Poland syndrome: description of two patients in the same family]. An Pediatr (Barc). 2008;69(1):49–51.
40. Fuhrmann W, Mösseler U, Neuss H. [Clinical and genetic aspects of Poland's syndrome]. Dtsch Med Wochenschr. 1971;96(25):1076–8.
41. Tomo I, Vrsanský V. [Contribution to the elucidation of potential teratogenic influences on the development of malformations of the upper extremities (author's transl)]. Bratisl Lek Listy. 1975;63(5):531–8.

Computer-Aided Design: Prototyping and Manufacturing (Pectus Excavatum and Poland Syndrome)

Benjamin Moreno, Pierre Leyx, and Jean-Pierre Chavoin

2.1 Introduction

Congenital malformations of the thorax are largely dominated by funnel chest, also known as Pectus Excavatum [1]. It is a complex malformation involving the sterno-costal plastron. It is characterized by a median depression with a large vertical axis, sometimes lateralized, touching the second part of the sternum, invaginating the cartilages from the third to the eighth coast [2] (Fig. 2.1). Scoliosis is often associated with thoracic deformity (Fig. 2.2).

Clinical forms of funnel chest have been the subject of several classifications. The classification of Chin [3] based on a series of 54 patients has the advantage of taking into account the degree of asymmetry that a funnel chest can present.

- Type I: It is a narrow and symmetrical deformation. The angulation of the costal cartilages is acute but does not exceed the mammary line (Fig. 2.3).
- Type II: The deformation, still symmetrical, is wider than the previous one and crosses the breast line. The inclination of the cartilages is gentle to the sternum (Fig. 2.4).
- Type III: These are asymmetric or unilateral deformations. The depression can be extended or localized, accompanied by a sternal rotation (Fig. 2.5).

Chest malformations are most often a physical disgrace without associated functional manifestations.

B. Moreno · P. Leyx
AnatomikModeling, 19 Rue Jean Mermoz, Toulouse, France
e-mail: bmoreno@anatomikmodeling.com; pleyx@anatomikmodeling.com

J.-P. Chavoin (✉)
Plastic Surgery Department, Rangueil Hospital, Toulouse University Hospital, Toulouse, France
e-mail: jean-pierre.chavoin@orange.fr

© Springer Nature Switzerland AG 2019   13
J.-P. Chavoin (ed.), *Pectus Excavatum and Poland Syndrome Surgery*,
https://doi.org/10.1007/978-3-030-05108-2_2

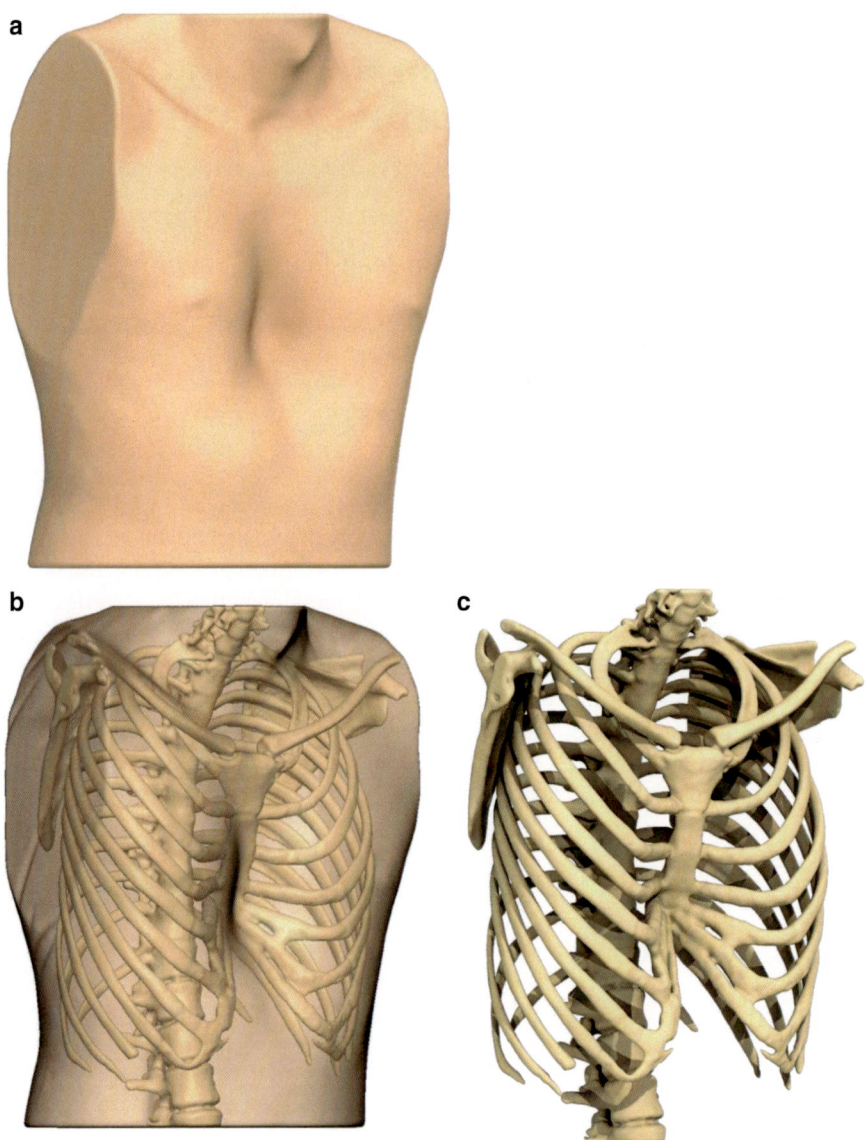

Fig. 2.1 Funnel chest (Pectus Excavatum) anatomical aspect. (**a**) Cutaneous plan. (**b**) Transparent skin, underlying bone plane. (**c**) Bony plan

Another type of congenital malformation of the thorax is Poland syndrome (Fig. 2.6). It is the association of two anomalies that defines this syndrome:

– Hypoplasia of the pectoralis major
– Malformation of the homolateral hand

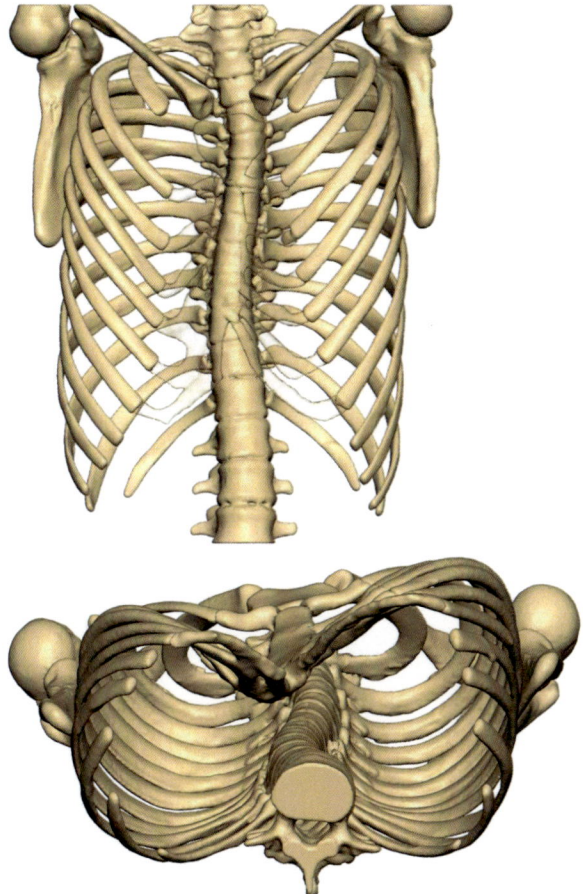

Fig. 2.2 Pectus Excavatum associated with scoliosis

Malformations vary from one case to another, but still have in common the agenesis of the sternocostal fascicles of the pectoralis major. For the majority of authors [4–6], agenesis affects both the lower and middle sternocostal beam, the clavicular beam being intact. However, some patients in our series also have agenesis of the clavicular beam. In this case, a complete agenesis of the pectoralis major and the pectoralis minor is noted (Fig. 2.7).

The correction of Pectus Excavatum malformations by radical surgical techniques of sternochondroplasty is heavy, the morbidity is not negligible, results are inconsistent, and recurrences are frequent. The aim of the intervention being therefore purely morphological or cosmetic, the correction by filling becomes logical. After a few unsuccessful attempts at autogenic filling, the unanimous supporters of the filling turned to silicone. The same reconstruction technique can be applied to the treatment of thoracic malformations of Poland syndrome, the aim of the treatment being purely aesthetic.

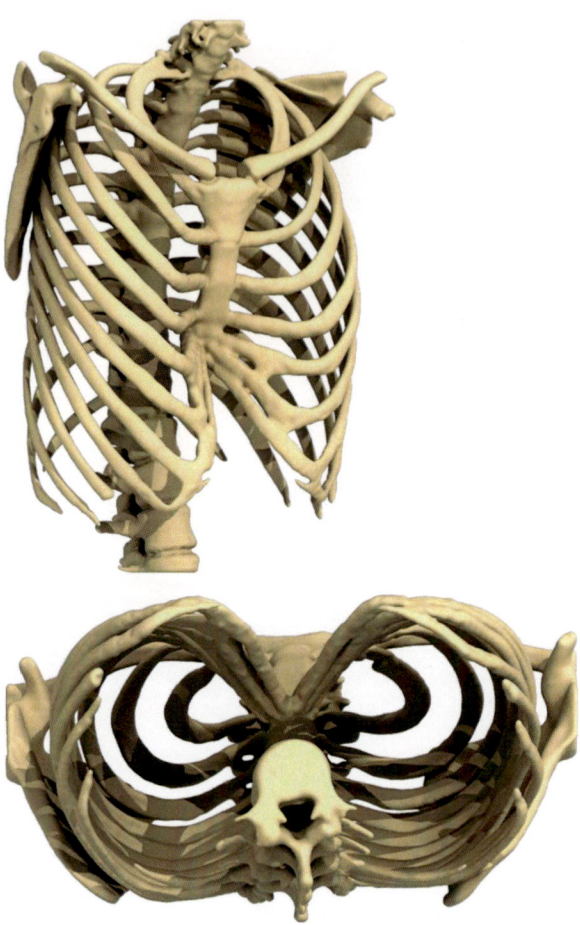

Fig. 2.3 Type I Pectus Excavatum, 3D reconstruction

Murray was the first in 1965 [7] to use a preformed silicone prosthesis, followed in the 1970s [8–12] by many other health professionals. The conventional technique consists in making the prosthesis in the laboratory, using a deformation imprint. The prosthesis is thus made in accordance with the visible deformation of the skin and not that of the surgical plane where it will be deposited. In women, the presence of the breast is an additional embarrassment to the appreciation of the deformity. Although refinements have been made to this method, ignorance of the thickness of the soft tissues leads to defects that sometimes make the prosthesis visible during postoperative treatment. The use of computer-aided design (CAD) of the implants based on a three-dimensional reconstruction of patient's thoracic scan allows to solve these appreciation issues.

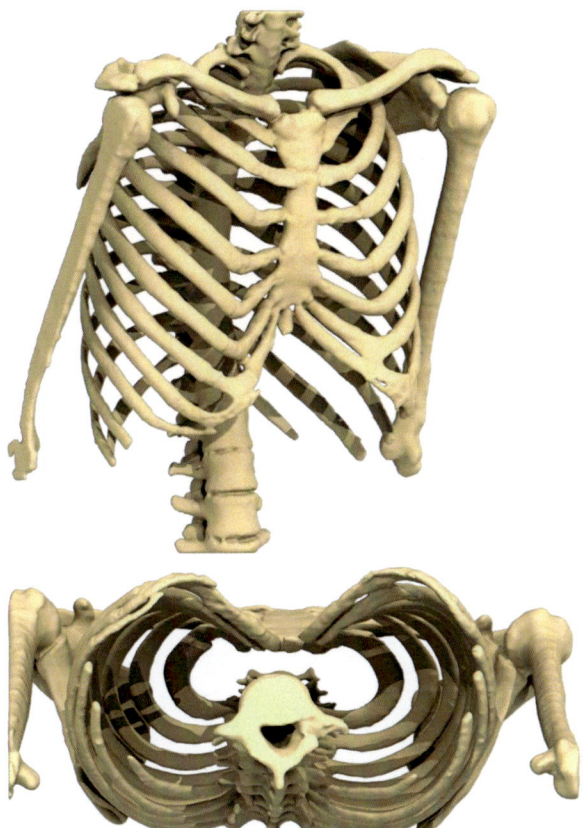

Fig. 2.4 Type II Pectus Excavatum, 3D reconstruction

2.2   Method

Computer-aided design (CAD) has for many years been widely used in the industry. After conquering many fields of activity, it found many applications in the medical field both for simulation and for CAD itself.

This is greatly facilitated by advances in medical imaging and signal processing. The evolution of CT scanning processes, marked by the advent of helical acquisition in 1989, allows high-quality multi-planar and three-dimensional reconstructions.

The preliminary to any treatment based on the use of CAD implants is thus the realization of a digitalized tomodensitometric examination, at the base of the 3D reconstruction, which is the support of the realization of the silicone implant (Fig. 2.8).

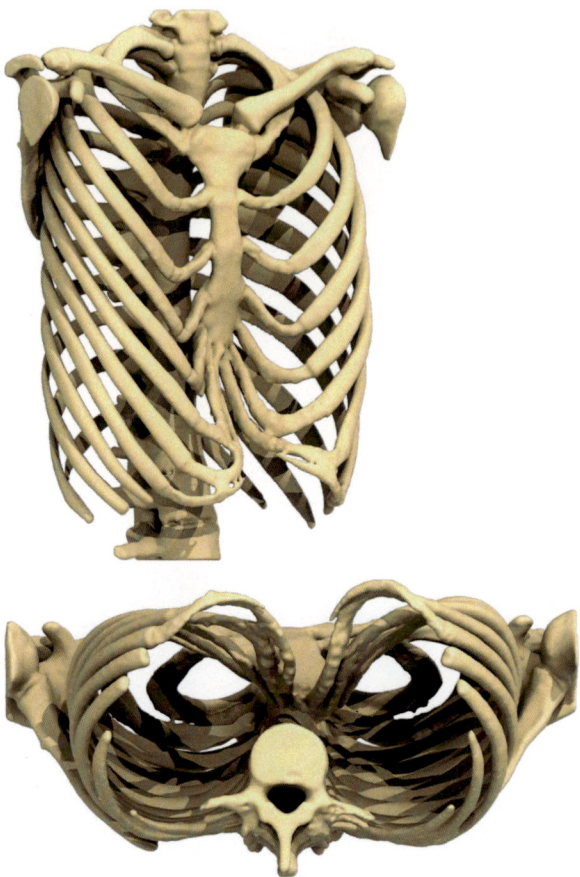

Fig. 2.5 Type III Pectus Excavatum, 3D reconstruction

A thoracic helical acquisition scanner in contiguous sections with a maximum thickness of 1–1.2 mm is necessary to obtain a precise three-dimensional model. No contrast agent is necessary. This CT scan has to be done with the arms along the body in supine position. Indeed, the arm-raised CT scan results in a significant deformation of the muscular position, which is detrimental to the design of the implant, especially in the case of Poland syndrome.

2.2.1　Computer-Assisted Design

Several computer processing steps occur during the computer-aided design of the prosthesis.

2.2.1.1 Three-Dimensional Reconstruction and Segmentation
The DICOM (Digital Imaging for Communication in Medicine) two-dimensional sections of the scanner are virtually re-stacked to obtain the three-dimensional model of patient's thorax.

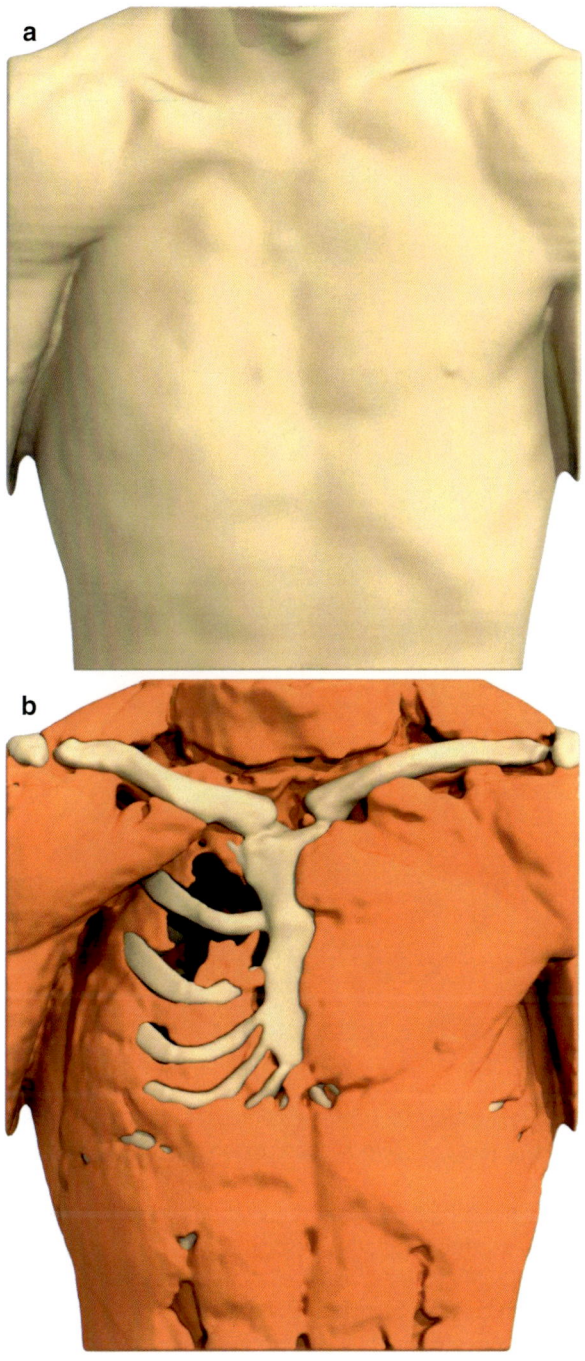

Fig. 2.6 Poland syndrome anatomical aspect. (**a**) Cutaneous plan. (**b**) Musculo-skeletal plan

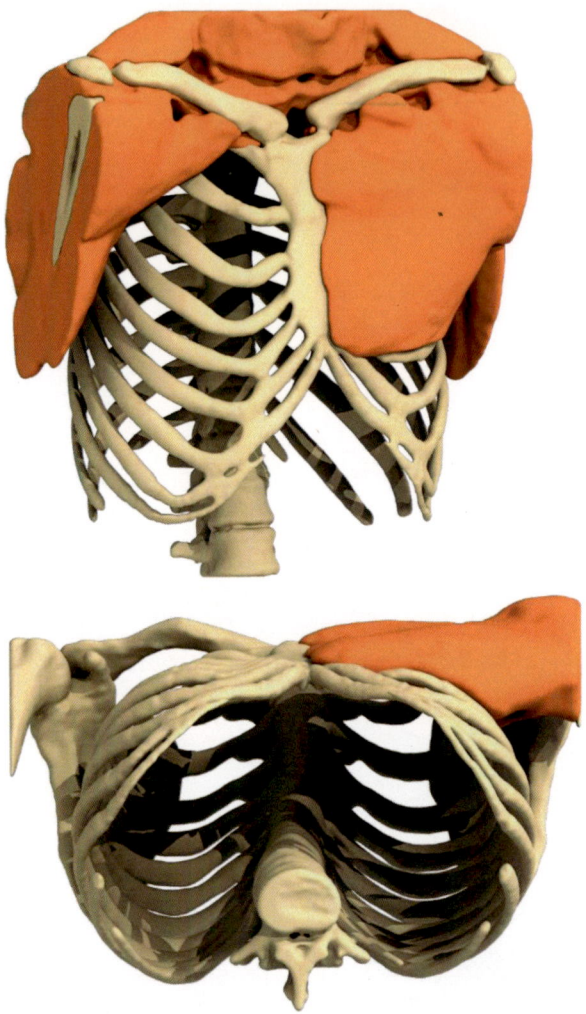

Fig. 2.7 Poland syndrome, 3D reconstruction

The different planes must then be segmented. Actually, it is to separate the bone and cartilage, muscular and skin planes, to obtain the three-dimensional virtual patient body.

Three 3D models are thus obtained representing, respectively, the bone and cartilage, the muscles and the cutaneous tissues.

2.2.1.2 Determination of Surgical Plan

The surgical plane is determined on the three-dimensional model. It is represented by a plane that exactly corresponds to the dorsal surface of the future implant.

7. Murray J. Correction of pectus excavatum by synthetic subcutaneous implant. Philadelphia: American Society of Plastic and Reconstructive Surgery; 1965.

8. Marks M, Argenta L, Lee D. Silicone implant correction of Pectus Excavatum: indications and refinement in technique. Plast Reconstr Surg. 1984;74:52–8.

9. Masson JK, Payne WS, Gonzalez JB. Pectus Excavatum: use of preformed prosthesis for correction in the adult. Plast Reconstr Surg. 1970;46(4):399.

10. Mendelson B, Masson JK. Silicone implants for contour deformities of the trunk. Plast Reconstr Surg. 1977;59(4):538–44.

11. Stanford W, Bowers DG, Lindberg EF, Armstrong RG, Finger ER, Dibbell DG. Silastic implants for correction of Pectus Excavatum: a new technique. Ann Thorac Surg. 1972;13(6):529–36.

12. Nordquist J, Svensson H, Johnsson M. Silastic implant for reconstruction of Pectus Excavatum: an update. Scand J Plast Reconstr Surg Hand Surg. 2001;35(1):65–9.

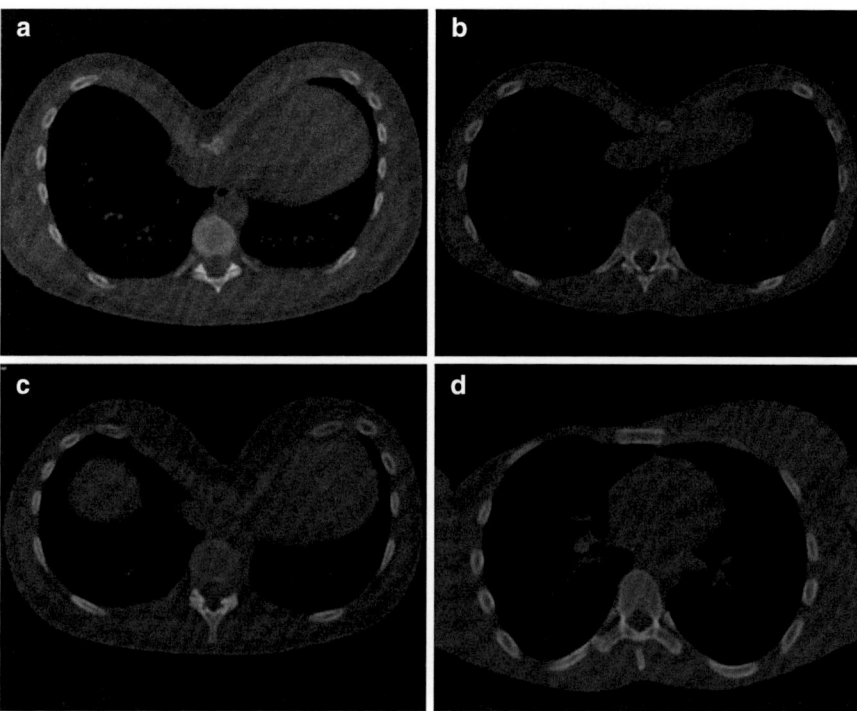

Fig. 2.8 Axial slices of CT exams. (**a–c**) Three cases of Pectus Excavatum. (**d**) One case of Poland Syndrome

In the case of a pectus excavatum, this plane includes the sternum, the intercostal muscles, and the right muscles of the abdomen. It excludes the small and large pectoral muscles (Figs. 2.9, 2.10, and 2.11).

In the context of a Poland syndrome, this plane includes the distal side, the sternum, and the sternoclavicular head of the pectoralis major (Figs. 2.12 and 2.13).

2.2.1.3 Implant Design
The implant is then 3D designed to give the ribcage a harmonious shape. The edges are refined to minimize the visibility of the implant. The thickness of the skin tissues overlying the prosthesis is known and taken into account in the elaboration of the latter. Studies are underway to perform a dynamic simulation of soft tissue deformation mimicking placement of the prosthesis on the virtual patient body.

In the case of a pectus excavatum, a sternal depression and an epigastric depression are sculpted on the ventral surface of the prosthesis (Figs. 2.13, 2.14, and 2.15).

In the case of a Poland syndrome, the cranial margin of the implant "espouses" the sternoclavicular head of the pectoralis major when it is present (Figs. 2.16 and 2.17).

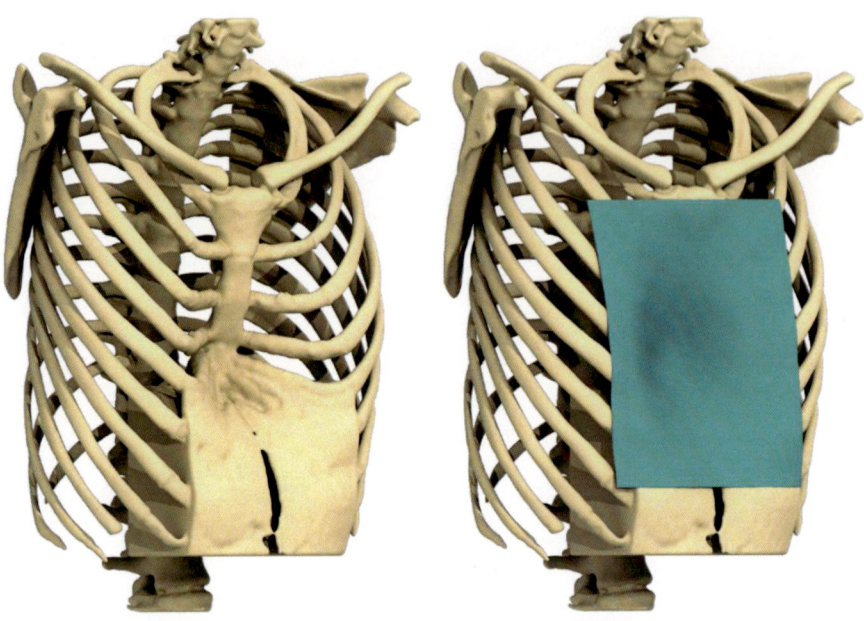

Fig. 2.9 Determination of the surgical plan in the case of a Type I Pectus Excavatum

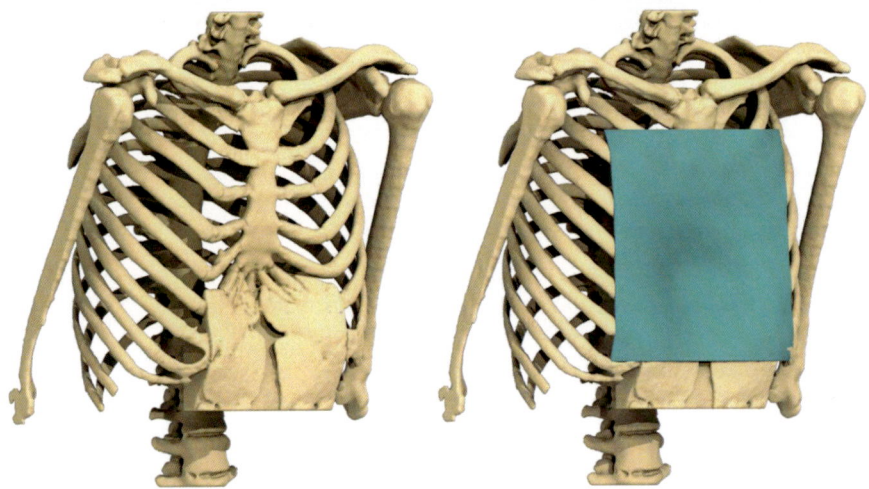

Fig. 2.10 Determination of the surgical plan in the case of a Type II Pectus Excavatum

2.2.2 Manufacturing of the Implant

Once the three-dimensional model of the implant is realized, a block of polyure-thane is machined at scale 1:1 by 3D CNC (Computer Numerical Control) machin-ing. This allows to obtain a physical positive model of the future implant.

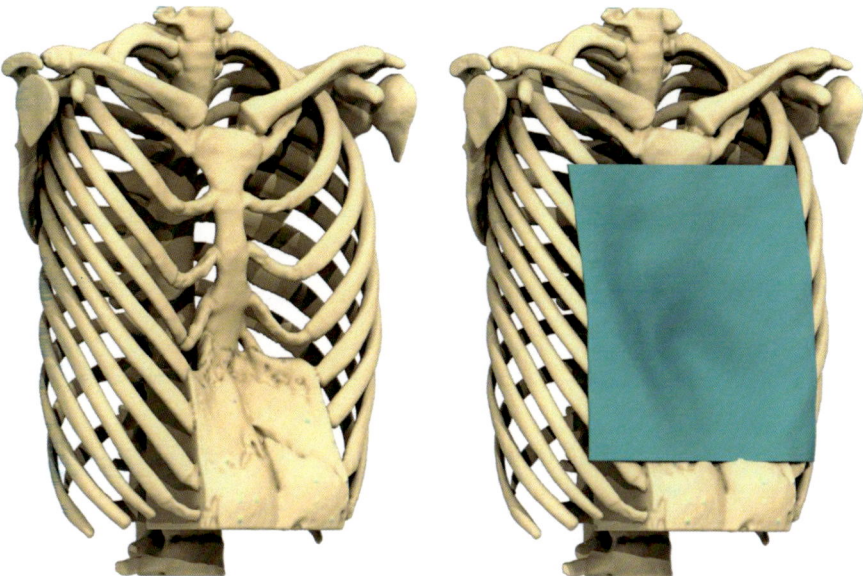

Fig. 2.11   Determination of the surgical plan in the case of a Type III Pectus Excavatum

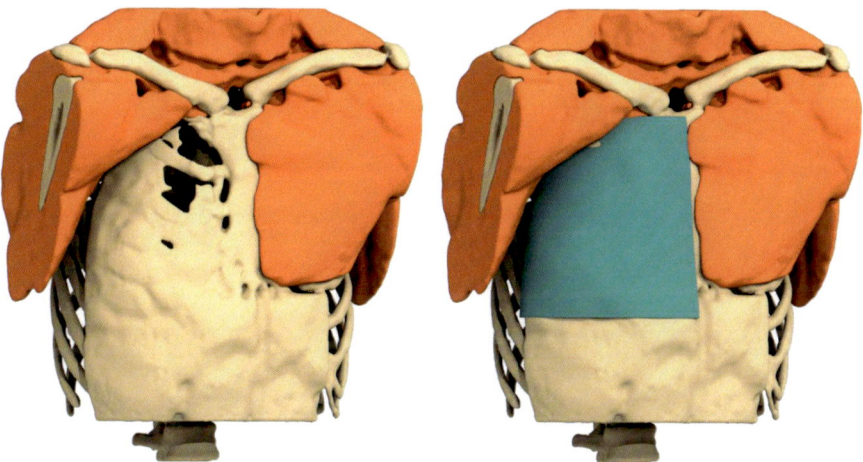

Fig. 2.12   Determination of the surgical plan in the case of a Poland syndrome

This step is necessary in order to be able to produce a plaster mould in the laboratory, which is a negative model of the prosthesis, which will be used for the casting of the long-term medical grade silicone. To do so, the prototype is coated with a release agent such as an aqueous solution of soap in order to make demoulding easier.

The silicone that is poured in the plaster mould is a silicone elastomer, as opposed to silicone gel for breast implants. Breast implants are made of a silicone elastomer

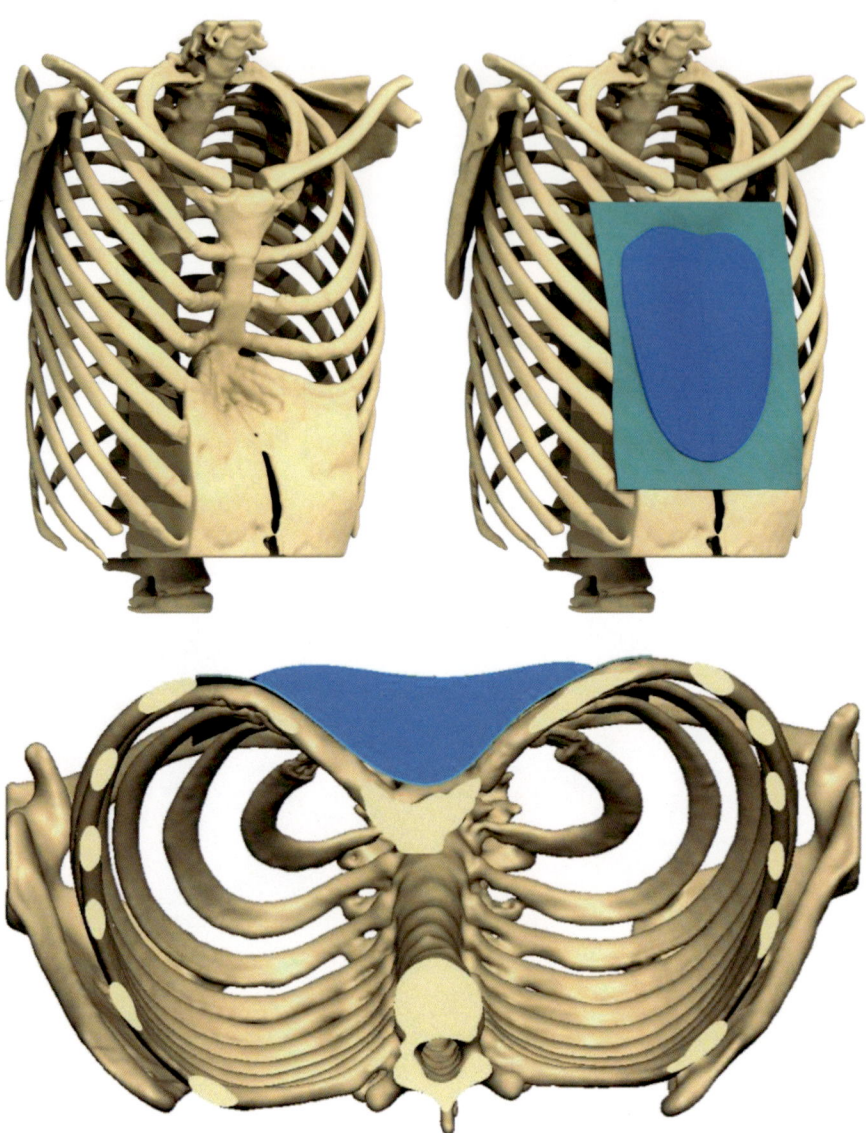

Fig. 2.13 Design of the prosthesis in the case of a Type I Pectus Excavatum

shell filled with cohesive silicone gel. Silicones, or PolySiloxanes for scientists, are inorganic polymers made up of repeating units of siloxane, which is a chain of alternating silicon atoms and oxygen atoms ($-Si-O-$)n, frequently combined with carbon and/or hydrogen. Some inorganic compounds can be used to link several of those polymeric chains together.

The most common silicone is PolyDiMethylSiloxane PDMS. Some common forms include silicone oil, silicone gel, or silicone elastomer/rubber depending on their physical states (viscosity, crosslinking percentage, mechanical properties).

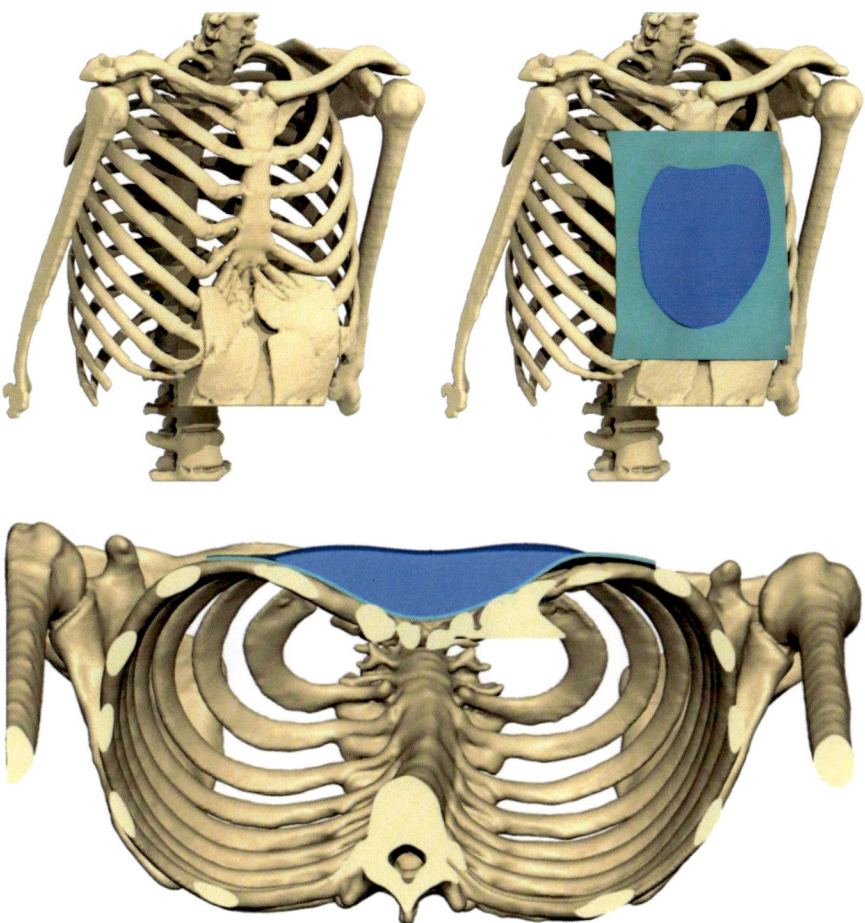

Fig. 2.14 Design of the prosthesis in the case of a Type II Pectus Excavatum

Moreover, mechanically speaking, the main difference between silicone gel and silicone rubber lies in the crosslinking percentage: silicone rubber is partially vulcanized/crosslinked while silicone gel is not. Silicone rubber consistency is that of a more or less flexible gum depending on the thickness and the indication, it is inalterable, unbreakable, and indestructible and cannot undergo retractable hull. Therefore, the final implant will be in place for life.

Polymerization is permitted by the addition of catalyst. In order to avoid the formation of air bubbles during the base-catalyst mixture, the latter is carried out under vacuum. The proportion of catalyst will determine the consistency of the implant, which should not be too hard or too soft and fragile.

The semi-rigid prosthesis obtained is then trimmed and finished.

Sterilization is carried out with ethylene oxide. EtO gas seeps into the packaging and at the very heart of the product to destroy the micro-organisms introduced during production or packaging operations. Then, it needs 2 weeks to let EtO gas degassing (Figs. 2.15b and 2.18).

2.2.3 Results

These implants are very well tolerated by patients who fully integrate them into their body regimen. The results are good, with significant patient satisfaction.

Patient's satisfaction for Pectus Excavatum is increased by 30% by using CAD 3D custom made implants versus traditional plaster moulding on the patient skin [1].

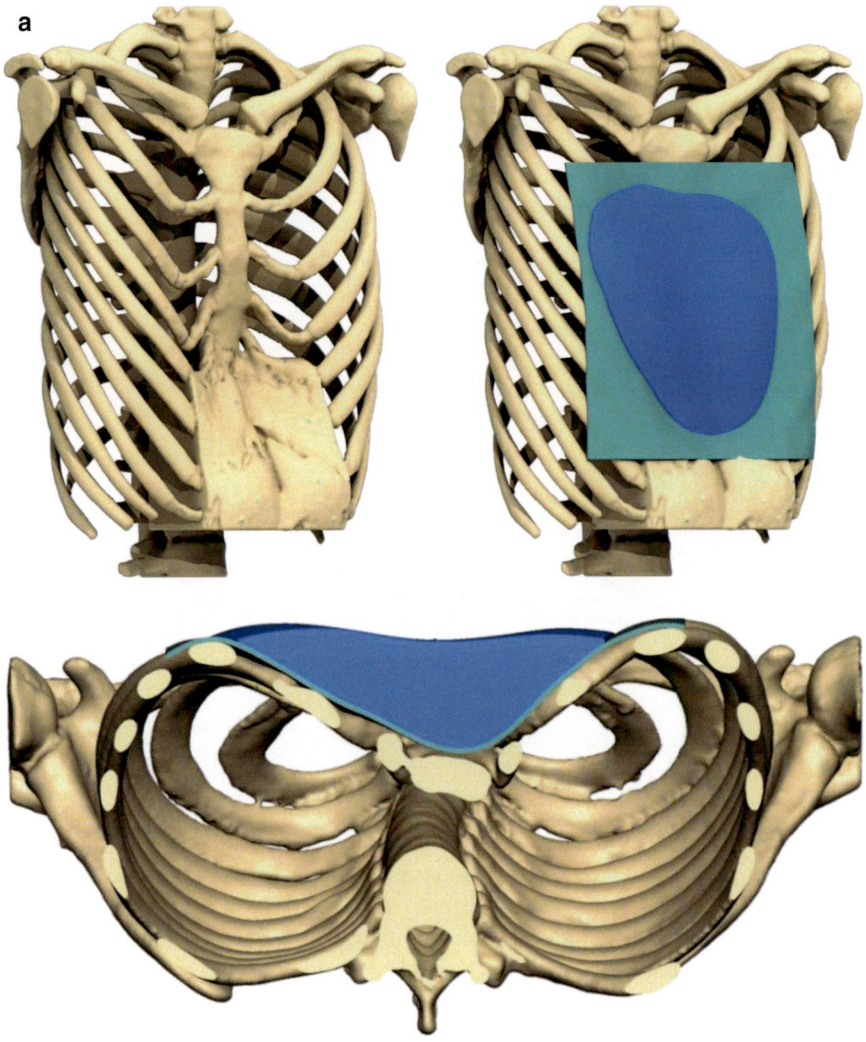

Fig. 2.15 Design of the prosthesis in the case of a Type III Pectus Excavatum. (**a**) Prosthesis in place. (**b**) Prosthesis details

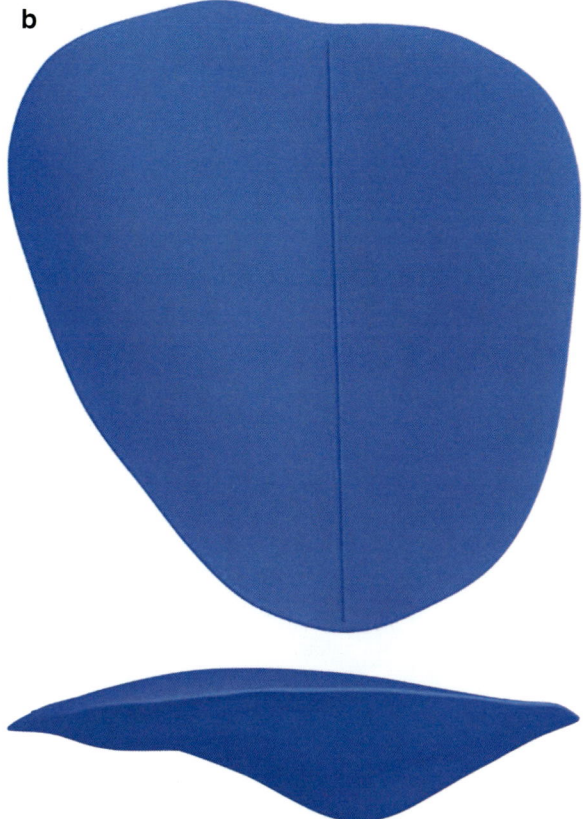

Fig. 2.15 (continued)

This is due to two main factors:

- First, the ability to design an implant that can be placed submuscular because the deep surgical plane can be determined avoiding visible edges and enhancing implant's stability over time.
- Second, the thickness of the implant can be adjusted to get back the symmetry of the thorax even for women where breasts represent one more tissue to take into account (Fig. 2.19).

For Poland syndrome, CAD provides more freedom of design giving the capability to take in charge the great morphological variability of this pathology, providing better results than traditional plaster moulding technique (Chavoin J.P. et al. Correcting Poland syndrome with a custom-made silicone implant: Contribution of 3D computer-aided design reconstruction. *Plast Reconstr Surg.*—accepted, to be published August 2018). However, Poland syndrome is more challenging than Pectus Excavatum because implants are placed subcutaneous and they cannot mimic the dynamic movement of the Pectoralis Major muscle.

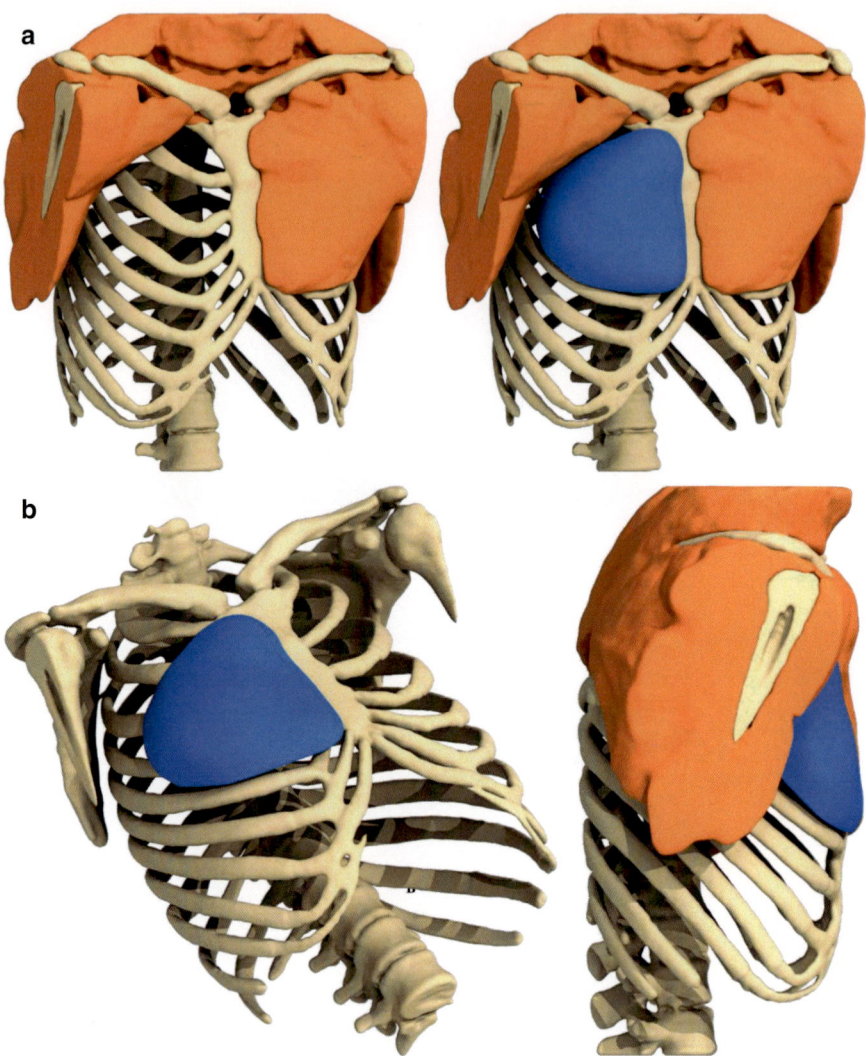

Fig. 2.16 (**a**, **b**) Design of the prosthesis in the case of a Poland Syndrome

2.3 Discussion

The two imperfections observed with the traditional moulding technique are the visibility of the prosthetic edges and the very flat aspect of the thorax. The common origin of these two pitfalls is the unknown thickness of the tissues covering the implant. Indeed, the impression of the thorax moulds the cutaneous deformation and not the chest deformation. Moreover, the production of prostheses by moulding technique is complex in women because of the presence of the breast around the deformation.

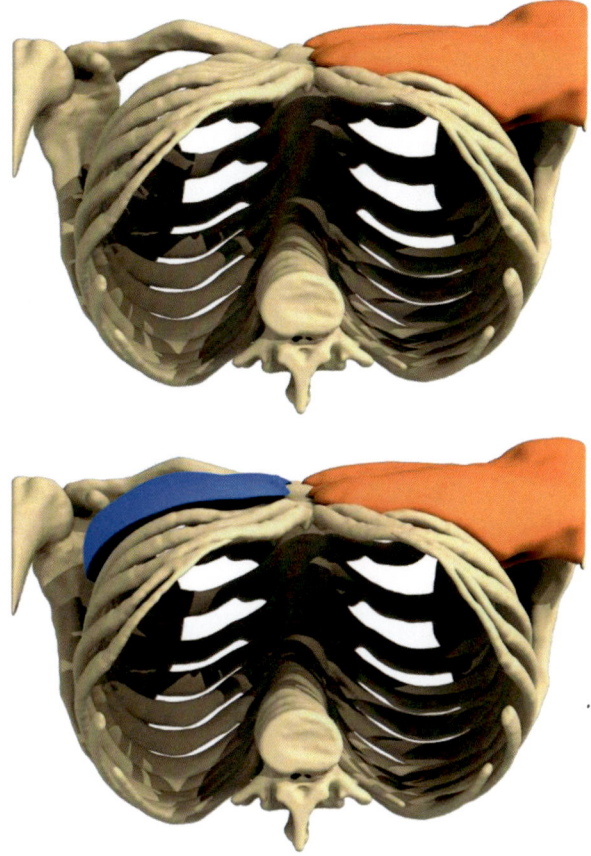

Fig. 2.17 Design of the prosthesis in the case of a Poland Syndrome, bottom views

In order to remove these pitfalls and improve the shape of the implant, the use of computer-aided design techniques has become established. The issue of the edges is solved by a precise modelling which perfectly matches with the edges of the surgical plane to avoid their protrusion. Knowledge of the thickness of the muscle and the skin, accurate at all points, allows precise modelling of the anterior surface of the implant to ensure a slight mid-thoracic depression. Finally, the computer-aided design of the implants makes it possible to give the latter a posterior face extremely faithful to the surgical plan on which it will rest. The implantation and the stability of the implant are thus considerably improved.

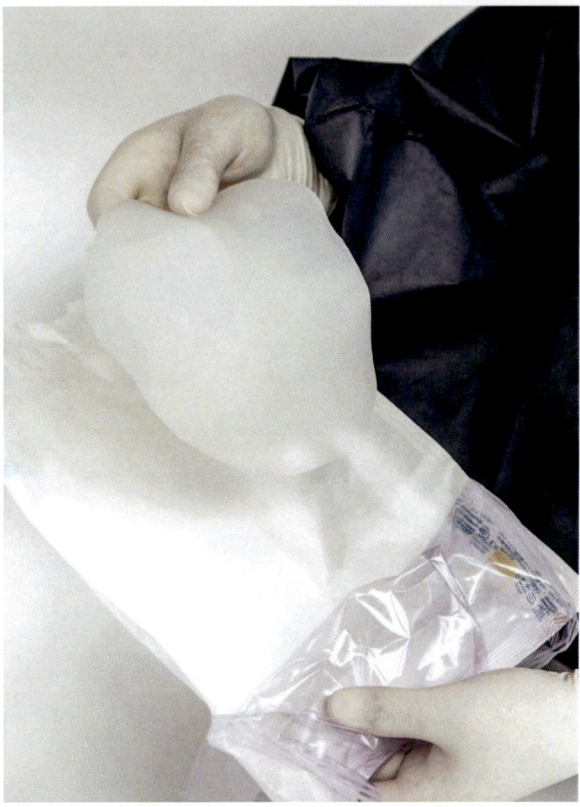

Fig. 2.18 Details of a prosthesis after manufacturing

2.4   Conclusion

The use of CAD to make implantable prostheses is nowadays the most appropriate technique. It allows the implant to be precisely adjusted to the anatomy of the patient, taking into account not only the surgical plan on which the prosthesis will rest, but also the thickness of the surrounding tissues.

This technique is applicable to the realization of implants made of silicone elastomer, intended for the correction by filling deformations but also in biocompatible materials other than silicone (polyetheretherketone (PEEK), etc.) for the design of prostheses for replacement of hard tissue (skull, zygomatic arch, etc.).

The evolution of computer science and current research will enable us to carry out simulations of deformations of the soft tissues after the installation of a prosthesis. A precise virtual visualization of the operative result will be possible as well as a control of the shape of the implant. The latter can therefore be reworked in such a way as to provide the best aesthetic result.

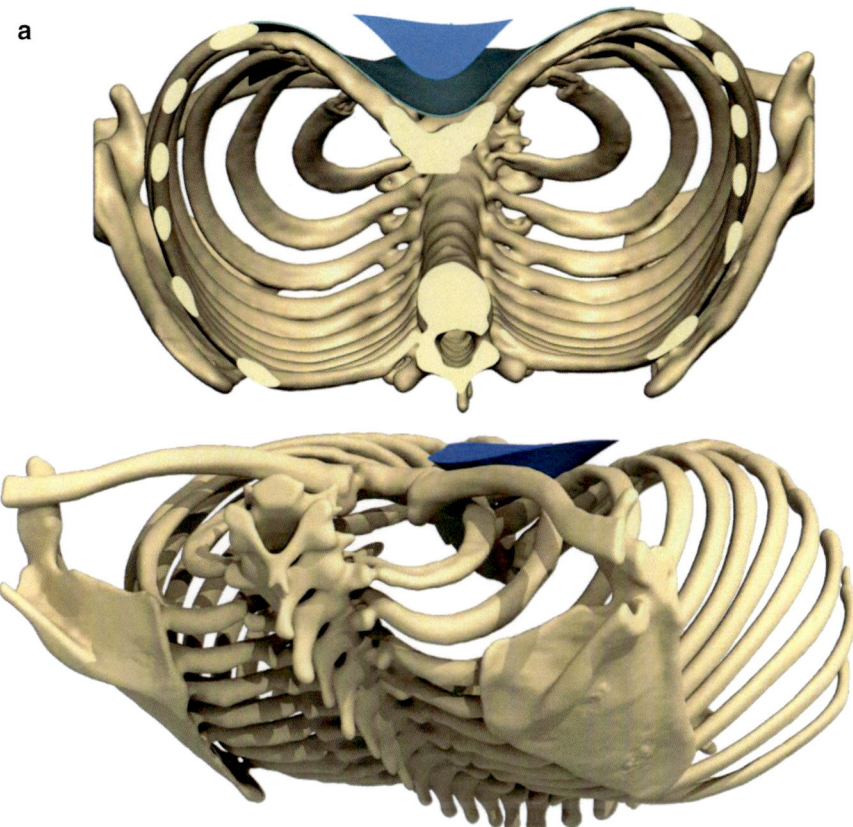

Fig. 2.19 Comparison of the adaptation between a prosthesis made by moulding and by CAD. (**a**) Prosthesis made by moulding, note the presence of dead spaces under-prosthetic. (**b**) Prosthesis made by CAD, note the adaptation of the prosthesis to the surgical plan

b

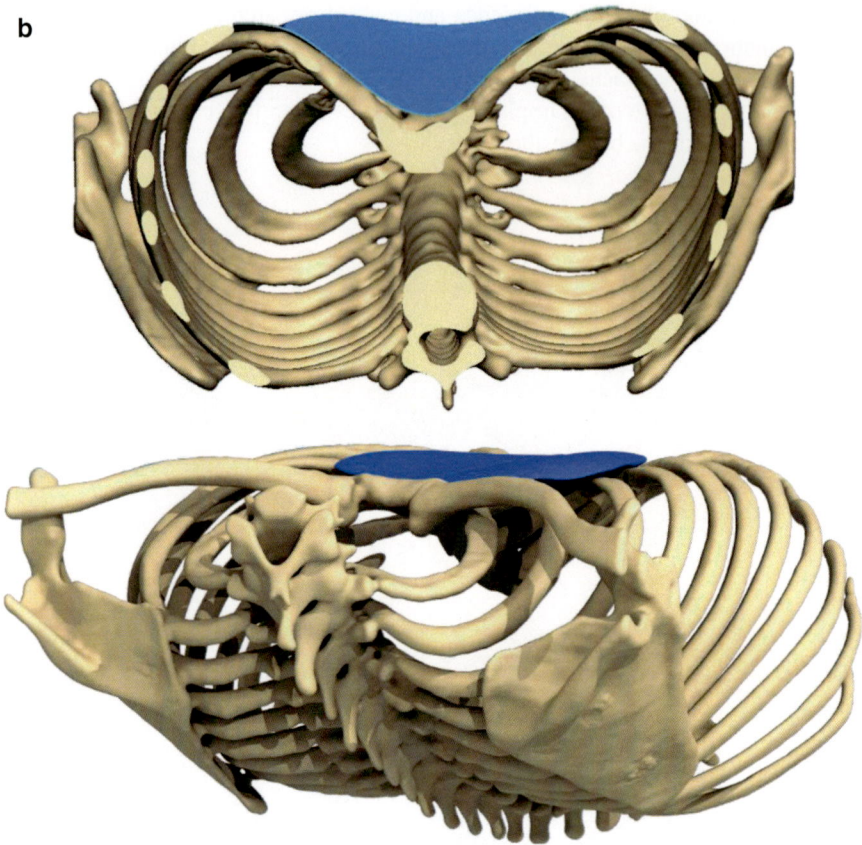

Fig. 2.19 (continued)

References

1. Chavoin J-P, Grolleau J-L, Moreno B, Brunello J, André A, Dahan M, et al. Correction of Pectus Excavatum by custom-made silicone implants: contribution of computer-aided design reconstruction. A 20-year experience and 401 cases. Plast Reconstr Surg. 2016;137(5):860e.
2. Chavoin JP, Dahan M, Grolleau JL, Soubirac L, Wagner A, Foucras L, et al. Funnel chest: filling technique with deep custom made implant. Ann Chir Plast Esthet. 2003;48(2):67–76.
3. Chavoin J, Grolleau J, Lavigne B, Darbas D, Dahan M, Pomard P. Chirurgie des malformations du thorax. Encycl Méd Chir. Techniques chirurgicales – Chirurgie plastique reconstructrice et esthétique. Paris: Elsevier; 1998. p. 45–671.
4. Chichery A, Jalibert F, Foucras L, Grolleau J, Chavoin J. Syndrome de Poland - EMC Techniques chirurgicales - Chirurgie plastique reconstructrice et esthétique; 2006. p. 17.
5. Fournier-Masse M, Castaing H, Fournet J, Glicenstein J, Duhamel B. Le syndrome de Poland. À propos de vingt observations. Ann Pediatr (Paris). 1976;23(4):285–92.
6. Pers M. Aplasias of the anterior Thoracic Wall, the pectoral muscles, and the breast. Scand J Plast Reconstr Surg. 1968;2(2):125–35.

7. Murray J. Correction of pectus excavatum by synthetic subcutaneous implant. Philadelphia: American Society of Plastic and Reconstructive Surgery; 1965.
8. Marks M, Argenta L, Lee D. Silicone implant correction of Pectus Excavatum: indications and refinement in technique. Plast Reconstr Surg. 1984;74:52–8.
9. Masson JK, Payne WS, Gonzalez JB. Pectus Excavatum: use of preformed prosthesis for correction in the adult. Plast Reconstr Surg. 1970;46(4):399.
10. Mendelson B, Masson JK. Silicone implants for contour deformities of the trunk. Plast Reconstr Surg. 1977;59(4):538–44.
11. Stanford W, Bowers DG, Lindberg EF, Armstrong RG, Finger ER, Dibbell DG. Silastic implants for correction of Pectus Excavatum: a new technique. Ann Thorac Surg. 1972;13(6):529–36.
12. Nordquist J, Svensson H, Johnsson M. Silastic implant for reconstruction of Pectus Excavatum: an update. Scand J Plast Reconstr Surg Hand Surg. 2001;35(1):65–9.

Pectus Excavatum Remodelling by CAD Custom-Made Silicone Implant: Experience of 600 Cases

3

Jean-Pierre Chavoin, Marcel Dahan, Benjamin Moreno, Jean-Louis Grolleau, and Benoit Chaput

3.1   Introduction

Pectus excavatum is the most common thoracic deformity, often familial [1]. The incidence thereof is 1/300 to 1/1000 births and the sex ratio 3:1 to 5:1 in the literature, 6:4 in our experience due to the success of women's and asymmetric case treatments. In the absence of any cardiac or respiratory impairment, the condition is a mere morphological deformation, but with a strong psychological impact for most of the authors [2–8].

The question of whether functional impairment can be present remains controversial [9–11]. There are only 15% of patients who are operated on [12], and the

Electronic Supplementary Material The online version of this chapter (https://doi.org/10.1007/978-3-030-05108-2_3) contains supplementary material, which is available to authorized users.

J.-P. Chavoin (✉) · J.-L. Grolleau · B. Chaput
Plastic Surgery Department, Rangueil Hospital, Toulouse University Hospital, Toulouse, France
e-mail: jean-pierre.chavoin@orange.fr; grolleau.jl@chu-toulouse.fr; chaput.b@chu-toulouse.fr

M. Dahan
Thoracic Surgery Department, Larrey Hospital, Toulouse University Hospital, Toulouse, France
e-mail: dahan.m@chu-toulouse.fr

B. Moreno
AnatomikModeling, 19 Rue Jean Mermoz, Toulouse, France
e-mail: bmoreno@anatomikmodeling.com

remaining 85% probably don't have cardiopulmonary problems to be treated. Despite this evidence, many thoracic and paediatric surgeons perform remodelling thoracic procedures such as the Nuss and Ravitch surgeries with interesting results [13–15], even for a confessed lifestyle surgery [16]. Recently developed, fat transfer techniques can be used in minor cases providing a significant improvement to patients, but in most deformations, limits of this treatment are quickly reached [17] due to the excessive volume to be corrected compared to the lack of fat in young patients.

Treatment of chest wall deformities remains challenging. Over 24 years (1993–2017), we have developed with thoracic surgeons' encouragements (M. Dahan) a true minimally invasive technique: we use permanent silicone elastomer custom-made implants. Initially (1993–2007), we manufactured prostheses using plaster moulds of the thorax [18], and later (2007–2017) employed computer-aided design (CAD) using 3D CT data [19].

To the best of our knowledge, no study has yet explored long-term satisfaction, quality-of-life (QOL), or cosmetic results, in so many patients [20].

We evaluated satisfaction and QOL using the questionnaire of Del Frari and Schwabegger [13] and the MOS-SF36. The evidence showed that CAD is far better than chest plaster moulding.

3.2   Patients and Methods

We include all (600) patients with pectus excavatum treated in our units of plastic and reconstructive surgery and thoracic surgery (Toulouse University Hospital, France) from January 1993 to March 2018. All patients were adults (14–64 yo), and all surgery was performed by the senior surgeon (J.P.C). No patients, even those with deep deformations, had any clinically relevant disorders (Haller index was on average 4.79 ± 2.33). This was confirmed by preoperative testing of ventilatory function (see Chap. 2). We confirmed the absence of comorbidities and researched associated malformations by clinical examination (Marfan or Poland syndrome, scoliosis, tuberous breasts, lateral slight pectus carinatum). The intrathoracic *Haller index* (defined by the ratio of the transverse diameter (horizontal distance inside the ribcage) and the anteroposterior diameter (shortest distance between the vertebrae and sternum)) served as a useful and informative measure of the severity of the condition, but is now completed with the *volume index* given by the computer-aided design. All possible thoracic reconstruction techniques are explained to each patient both orally and through information sheets.

Patients were classified from Type 1 to Type 3 according to the CHIN classification (1954 [21]), taking into account their anatomical shape. We added to this CHIN classification Type 4 for arcuatum and mixt asymmetrical mild carinatum and excavatum and Type 5 for secondary procedures after any type of primary treatment or traumatism. (Type 6 Hybrid associated with Poland syndrome, tuberous breasts, or other very rare associated genetic anomalies (Marfan, Turner, etc.)).

3.2.1   First Consultation: Patient's Information, Information Support, and Consent

- The patient is already thoroughly informed on the web and forums about the different surgical procedures.
  - Either with invasive orthopaedic techniques which tend to correct the chest's shape and are supposed to improve their functional problems due to a lung or heart disease.
  - Or with an implant to correct a morphologic anomaly and its psychological heavy consequences on the quality of their life.
- The consultant gives the patient oral information and documents to be read.
- A quotation is given for all the procedures:
  - Hospitalization's price
  - Custom-made implant price by the manufacturer
  - Surgeon's fees
- After the first oral agreement, a hand-written informed consent is sent by the patient.
- A complete functional exploration can be prescribed with:
  - Respiratory function exploration by plethysmography
  - CO alveolar-capillary transfer capacity
  - VO_2 max: O_2 consumption on cyclo-ergometer
  - Diaphragmatic function
  - Echocardiography standard or with stress

3.2.2   Custom-Made Implants via Computer-Aided Design

Several steps required are precisely described in the recommendations to the referent surgeons.

- Obtain a CT scan with 1–1.2 mm sections to get a good definition for 3D reconstruction and separate segmentations of different tissues: bone, cartilage, muscles, and skin.
- A computer scientist reconstructs the missing space between:
  - The deep plane, termed the "surgical plane" (ribcage, intercostal spaces, and sternum), which is reconstructed very accurately
  - The superficial plane (termed the "anatomical plane") which seeks (when necessary) to correct virtually symmetrical deformations and female breast's position
- The company *AnatomikModeling*® *SAS* performs the computer modelling and sends the images to the referent surgeon to get his agreement or corrections, so he becomes the real and responsible ***implant's designer***.
- Prototyping: A virtual image is subjected to 3D prototyping to make a polymer form.
- The implant prototype is performed by 3D CNC mills (computerized numerical control) by *AnatomikModeling*® *SAS*.

- Each implant is made from the prototype by a silicone implant manufacturer (Sebbin®, Boissy l'Aillerie, France) using a medical silicone elastomer (Nusil) by moulding and casting. The implant is semi-rigid and tear resistant. The implant is gas-sterilized next. Such implants are retained for the rest of the patient's life if the result is good.

3.2.3 Surgical Technique (Fig. 3.1)

Under general anaesthesia, the patient is placed supine, with the arms along the thorax. We routinely prescribe intraoperative prophylactic antibiotics (2 g of intravenous cefazolin injected when we start the surgery).

– *Preoperative drawings*: The prototype is placed on the thorax to check on the centreline positioning and its height precisely given by the distance between the sternal fork and the implant's distal limit as presented by the computer design (Fig. 3.2). We trace the perimeter of the implant with the prototype thus defining the precise limits of prosthetic placement (Fig. 3.3).

Fig. 3.1 Drawings of the procedure

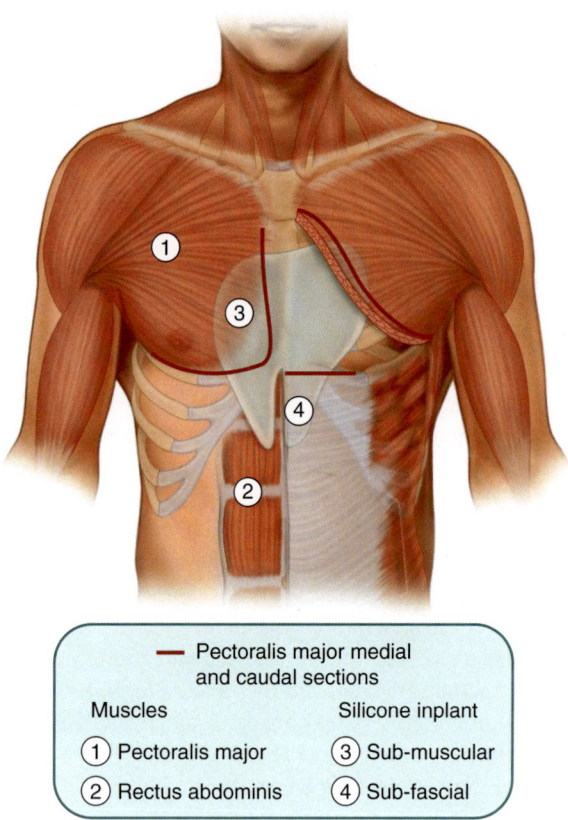

Pectoralis major medial and caudal sections

Muscles   Silicone inplant

① Pectoralis major   ③ Sub-muscular

② Rectus abdominis   ④ Sub-fascial

Fig. 3.2 Frontal implant's digital image with vertical distance

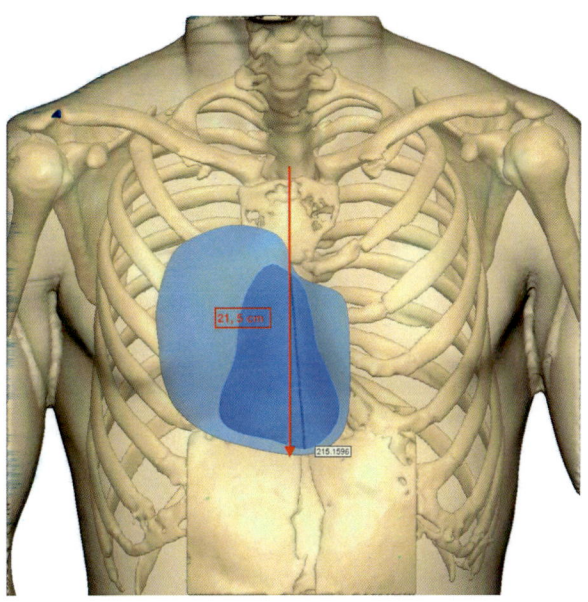

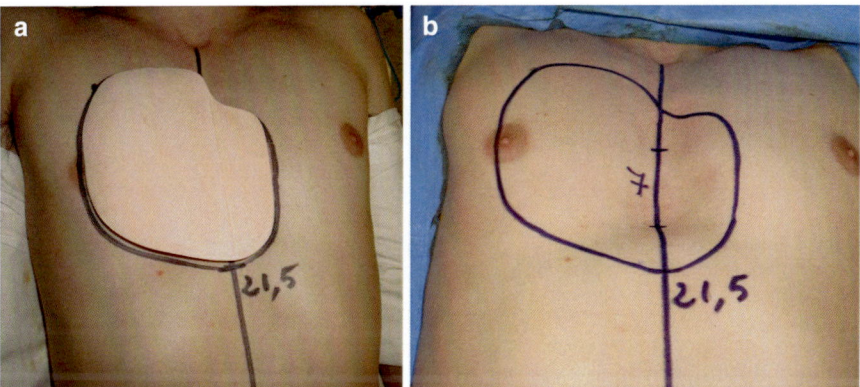

Fig. 3.3 (**a, b**) The implant's perimeter is traced with the prototype at the good height following the central line

– *Incision, dissection*: A vertical presternal incision of 6–8 cm is made in the centre of the deformation. Section continues until the sternal plane is attained. A bilateral medial detachment of the pectoralis major muscle is done, and then the submuscular undermining continues to the limits drawn on the chest skin. Medial perforating vessels are carefully coagulated. We use a front-head lamp and retractors (Fig. 3.4). The submuscular deep placement of implant's edges renders the implant undetectable both in vision and in touch.

The semi-rigid consistency of the implant makes bending and insertion thereof using a minimally invasive approach easy. These implants are easily foldable but not deformable and tearable (Fig. 3.5). The midline of the anterior implant's surface is

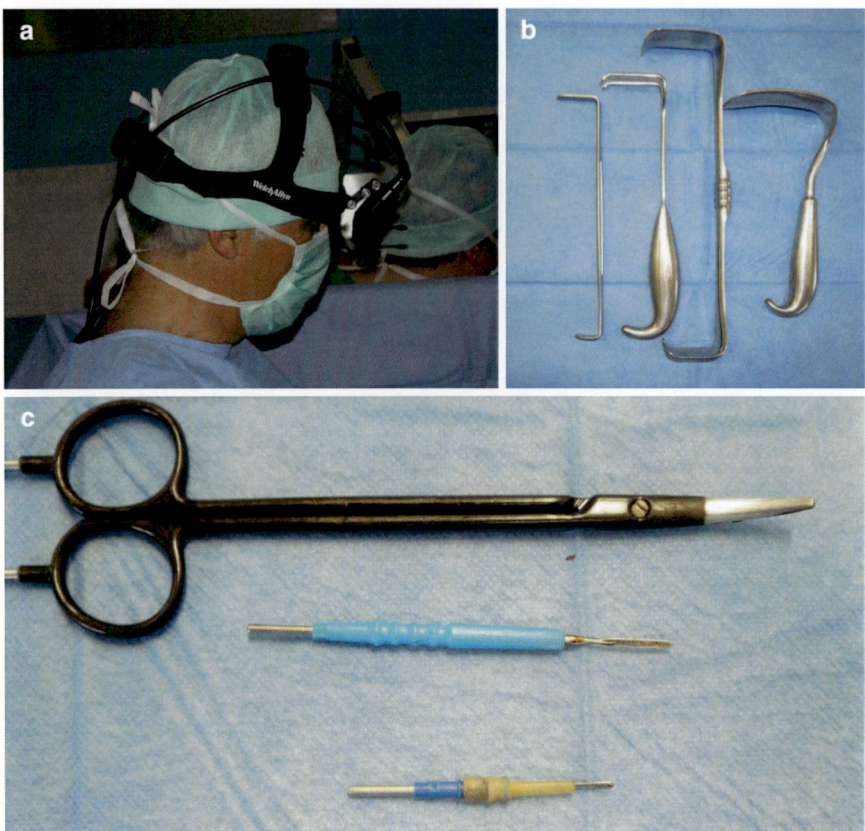

Fig. 3.4 (**a**) Front-head lamp. (**b**) Different types of retractors can be used: Kallmorgen, Richardson, Ollier, American (right to left). (**c**) Bipolar scissors and protected monopolar electric knife

marked by a line, which is used to correct any positional error and confirm the absence of rotation. The posterior face of the implant and prototype is marked with initials of name, surname, distance from the sternal fork and caudal limit, and proximal orientation. The implant takes easily a good position as its posterior face is perfectly adapted to the deep "surgical plane" with a stabilizing suction effect. The caudal end pole is cut 2–3 cm on the middle line and inserted subfascially, overlapping with the rectus abdominis intermuscular wall (Fig. 3.6).

This optimally stabilizes the implant, eliminating any risk of secondary displacement or rotation.

– *Closure features three steps*:
    Deep medial suturing of pectoralis major on the 2/3 cranial and deep fascia on the 1/3 caudal (Vicryl 0 big needle) (Fig. 3.7)
    Subcutaneous closure with reversed points (Monocryl 3/0)

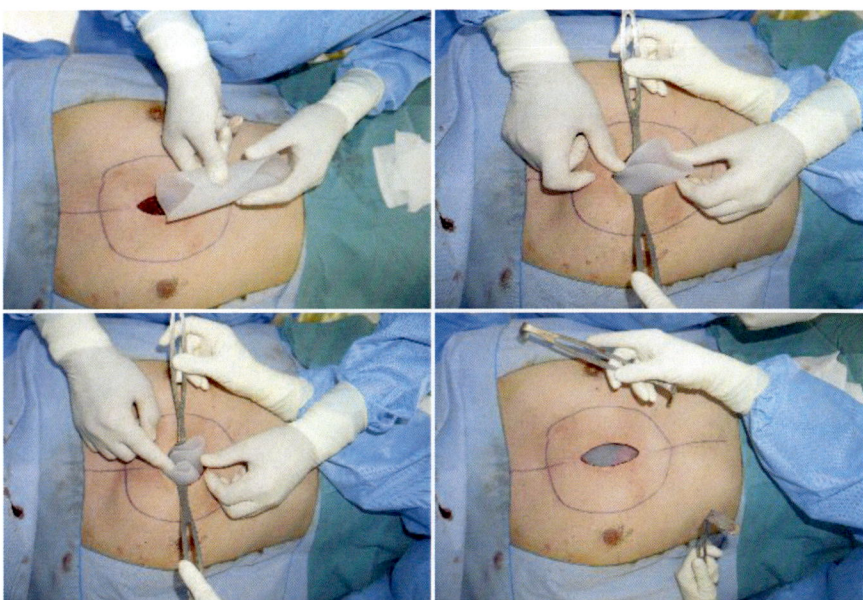

Fig. 3.5 Soft implant's insertion in submuscular position

Fig. 3.6 Caudal implant's
end is cut and overlaps the
intermuscular wall of
rectus abdominis, under its
anterior sheath

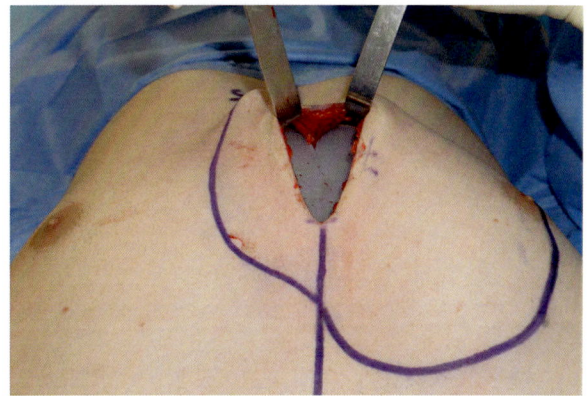

Skin closure via continuous intradermal suturing (Monocryl 3/0). **We do not
place suction drain anylonger,** but a medial circular contention (abdominal elastane belt thuasne® cicaflex) with a pressure garment (soft rolled Rolta® Dacron
band) (Fig. 3.8)

After 1 or 2 days, primary contention and dressing are taken off; most of the time
there is a sero-hematic collection under the skin and muscle in front of the smooth
implant: a first puncture is done in a half-seated position in the lower part, laterally
from the end side of the scar (19G needle and 60cc Luer-Lock syringe) (Fig. 3.9).

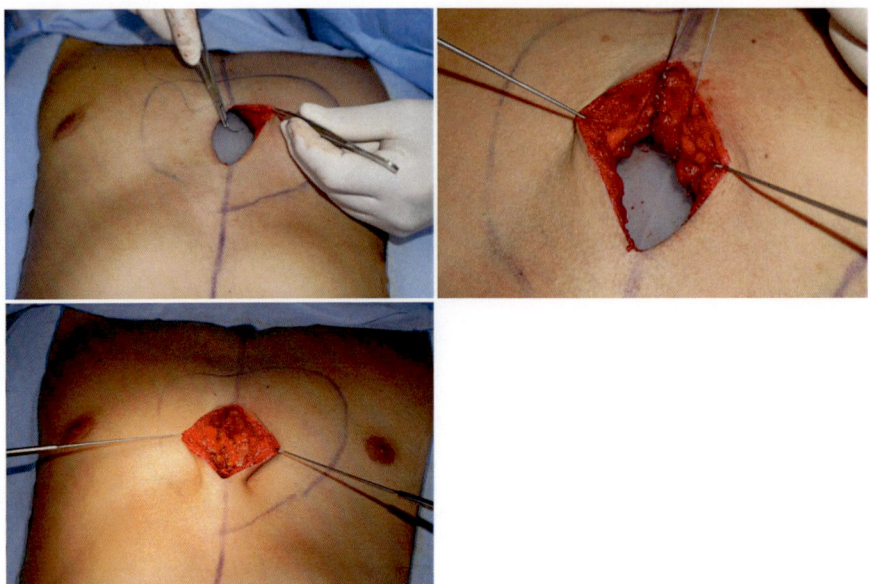

Fig. 3.7 Deep medial suturing of the two pectoralis major on the middle line

Fig. 3.8 Immediate
post-operative contention
with light elastane belt on
a soft Dacron felt rolled
band

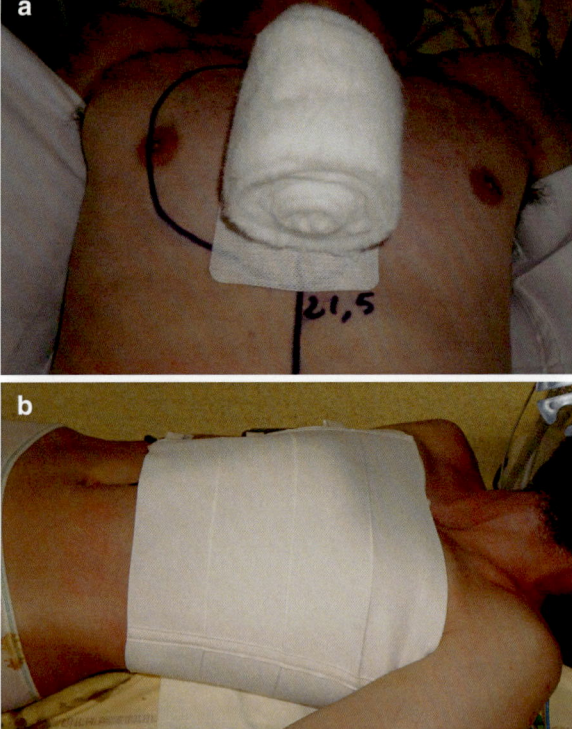

Fig. 3.9 Seroma's first
puncture in a half-seated
position

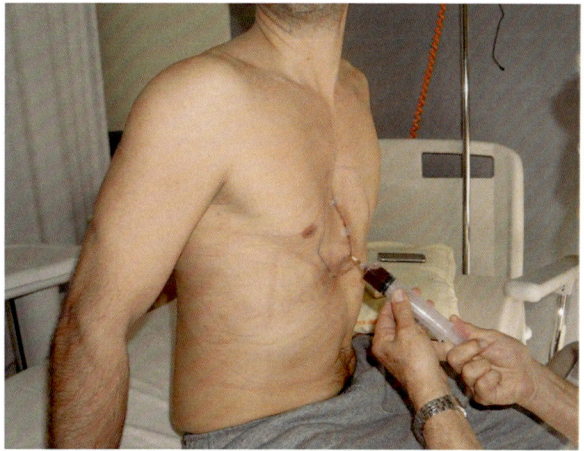

Fig. 3.10 Post-operative
brace with a pad is
indicated for 1 month 24/7

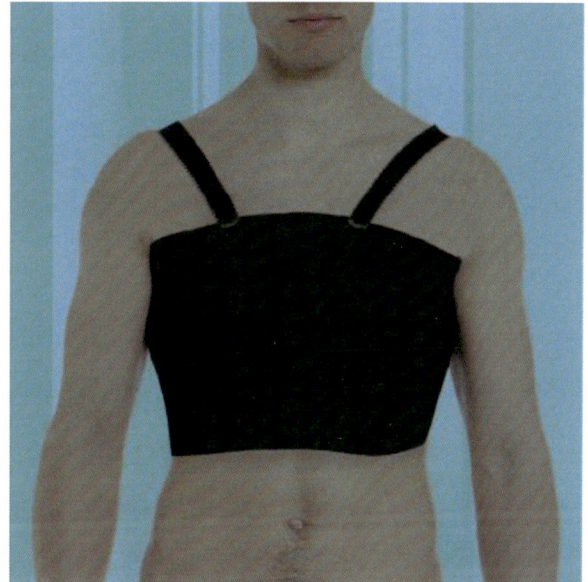

The puncture obtains between 5 and 200 cc of a sero-hematic collection, and then a new contention is put with a chest brace (medical Z® thoracic belt S33 and a smooth custom-made pad) (Fig. 3.10). The patient can go out with analgesic prescription (paracetamol 500 mg ×2 three times a day for 1 week).

If the puncture is not efficient with the needle due to fibrin obstruction, one can use a lipofilling cannula, through the cranial end of the scar under local anaesthesia in a half-seated position.

The dressing (mepilex border em ® style) is not changed for 1 week. Shower is recommended each day.

Eight days after, during the first consultation, a second seroma puncture in the sitting position is performed. Most patients return to work after 2 weeks.

The pressure brace and pad are kept for 1 month 24/7. Exercise cessation is recommended for 3 months due to the sutured muscle's vulnerability during that time. Afterwards any sport or physical activity can be played.

3.3   Results

We have treated consecutively 600 patients over a period of 25 years (1993–2017). The sex ratio was 1.43. The mean patient age was 27 years (14.9–55.5 years). The chin type 1 malformation was the most common in men (Fig 3.11) and chin type 3 in women (Fig. 3.12).

Implants are the best or the only indication of pectus excavatum type 3 in women and men (Figs. 3.13 and 3.14) and in athletic men (Fig. 3.15) and of pectus arcuatum in males (Fig. 3.16).

The operative time was about 1 h (45′ to 75′) for any type.

Overall, complications were very rare:

– We encountered only one **_infection_** on a secondary case after two failures, first with the Nuss and then the Ravitch technique with broken bar in two levels. The implant and the undermined space were largely washed and the implant was put

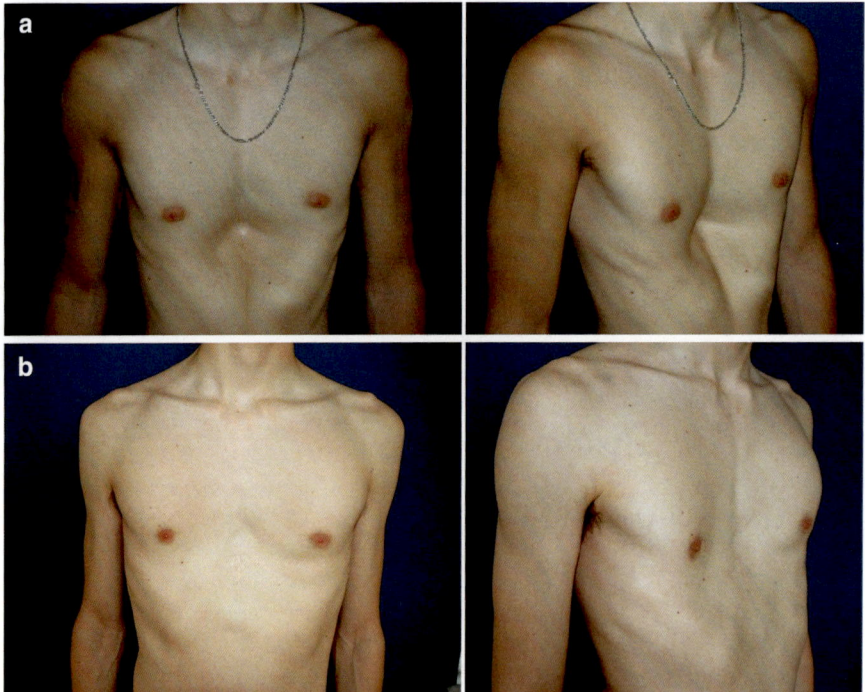

Fig. 3.11 Pectus excavatum type 1 in a man (**a**) before, (**b**) 1 year later

back in the same place, 10 days adapted antibiotherapy (M. sensitive staphylo-coccus), without following problem.

- Four *hematomas*: two due to a mistake with anticoagulant prescription, one due to an early trauma at 15 days post-op, and one due to a perforating vessel bleeding.
- Two cases of post-operative *wound dehiscence* due to a slight neglected electrical knife burn of the skin edges. It was managed by re-intervention (suture repair).
- All patients developed post-operative *seroma* completely managed by three transcutaneous punctures [1–5], as also reported by Wechselberger et al., despite drainage in 65% of patients [28].

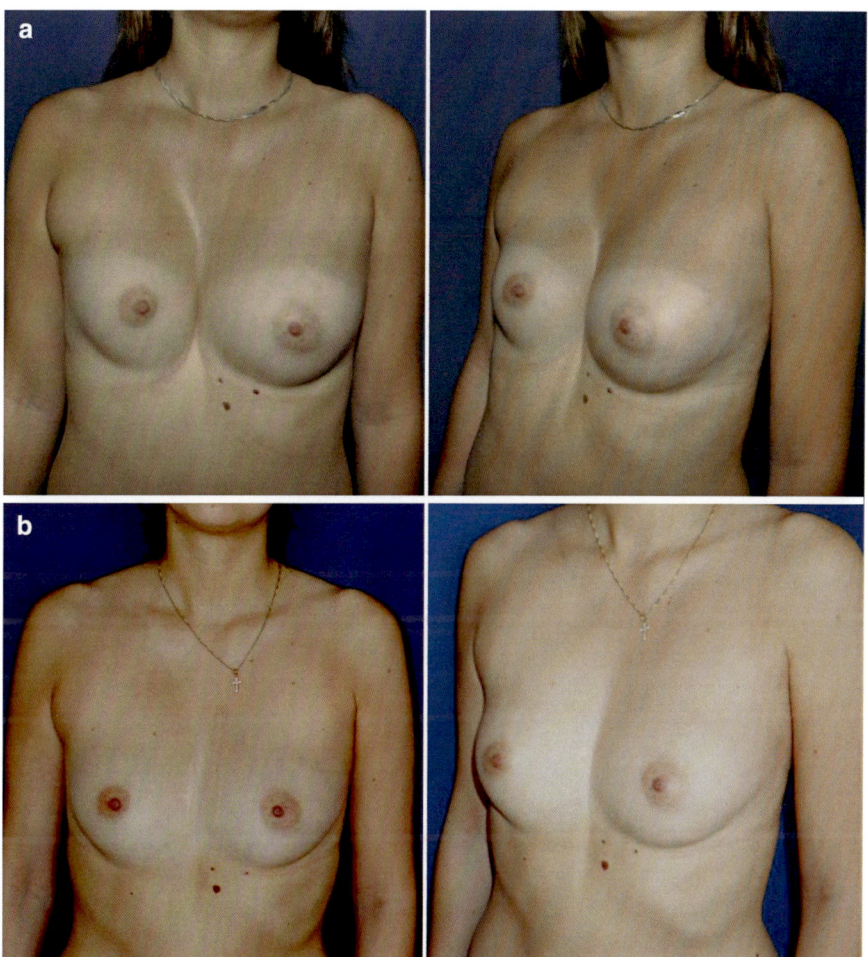

Fig. 3.12 Pectus excavatum type 3 in a woman: (**a**) before, (**b**) 1 year later, (**c**) CAD front face, (**d**) CAD supine

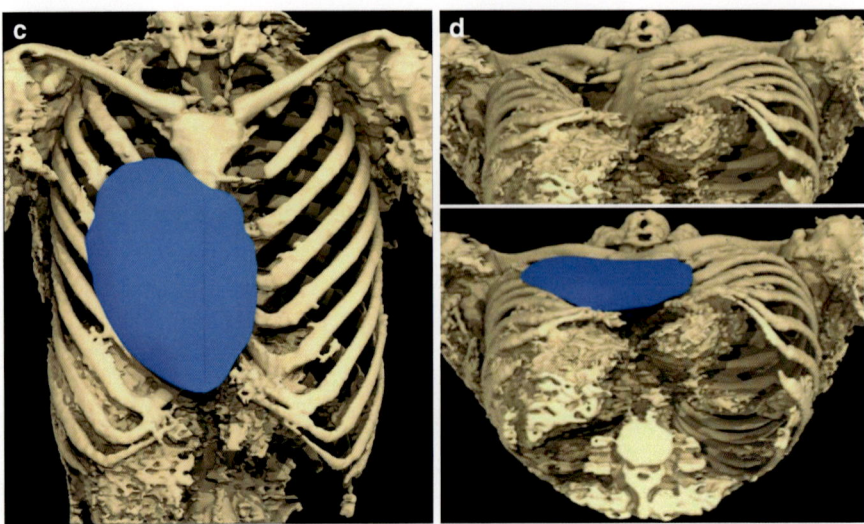

Fig. 3.12 (continued)

- All patients have a lack of cutaneous sensibility in the implant's area with a centripetal progressive recovering after 1 year.
- Two cases of implant's *rotation* had to be revised.
- We never have had any *capsular contracture* as it can be seen with round silicone gel breast implants.
- We never noticed *rupture or tearing* of these silicone elastomer implants.

In terms of satisfaction, 80% of patients reconstructed with the help of CAD were satisfied or very satisfied (scores 4 and 5). QOL assessed by the MOS-SF36 revealed significant improvement in "social functioning" and "emotional role" [20].

Some patients describe discomfort during intense sport practice, but without any pain quantifiable on a visual analogue scale. Most other MOS-SF36 items improved after placement of the prosthesis, but statistical significance was not attained.

3.4   Discussion

The use of custom-made silicone implants has been reported for the first time in 1965 by Murray [22], a plastic surgeon. Few thoracic surgeons used this procedure. The first was Toty [23] and then Dahan [18, 19], who had been with us since the beginning; Marks was the first to put the implants in a submuscular position [24]. The study of Johnson [25] is the only available in the literature using CT scans to design implants for three pectus excavatum. In this study, the patients showed excellent results. All other authors had short series of cases using plaster moulded and subcutaneously-placed implant after Mendelson in 1977 [26]. Nordquist et al. [27]

were the first in 2001 to report on pectus excavatum repair using silicone implants in a large series of patients. Almost 80% reported improvements in appearance and well-being. In In the same year, Wechselberger et al. [28] reported on a series of 20 patients, 90% of whom enjoyed good-to-excellent outcomes, and 10% acceptable results. In 2005, Margulis et al. [29] reported excellent corrections in a small series of seven patients compared with Horch [30] and Poupon [31]. More recently, in 2009, Snel reported that 83% of 16 patients were satisfied, and 69% considered their aesthetic outcomes to be good to excellent [32]. However, none of these authors employed CAD using 3D CT data.

The quasi-constant good results of our procedure are certainly due to CAD custom-made implants and their submusculofascial position [18–20].

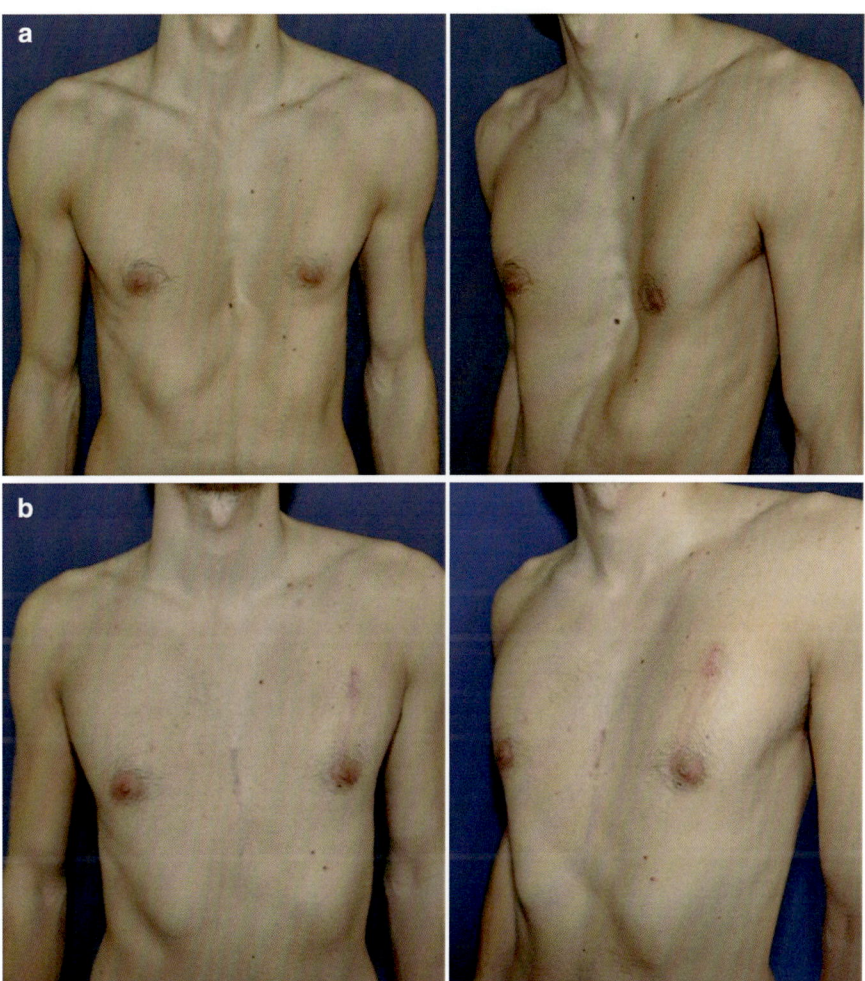

Fig. 3.13 Pectus excavatum type 3 in a man: (**a**) before, (**b**) 1 year later, (**c**) CAD front face, (**d**) CAD supine

Fig. 3.13 (continued)

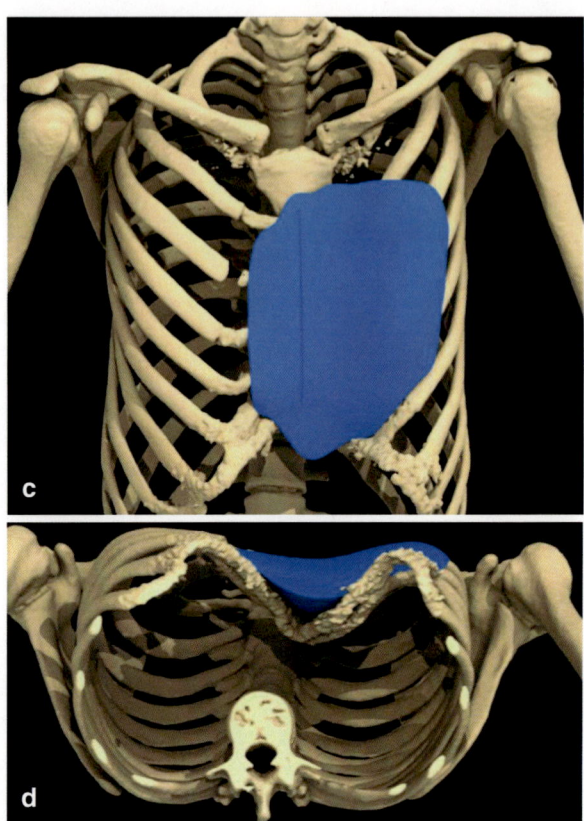

The extent of functional impairment associated with pectus excavatum remains highly controversial. Indeed, the recent meta-analyses of Malek et al. [10] and Guntheroth [11] on the pulmonary and cardiac consequences reveal that evidence bearing on any improvements in such conditions after thoracic surgery to correct malformations is lacking. In fact, such surgeries are cumbersome, and most patients (both adolescents and adults) seek only aesthetic and psychological relief [33–36].

Thus, we developed a reconstruction procedure prioritizing the cosmetic need. External suction systems are restricted to young patients and have not been always successful for adults [37, 38]. Fat tissue transfers (which can yield excellent results) require discrete shaping [17, 39]. Our technique is minimally invasive, easy, rapid, and associated with very low morbidity. In general, our surgical procedure takes less than 1 h and the hospital stay is less than 4 days. Most patients obtained satisfactory or very satisfactory aesthetic results [20].

The mean patient age was 27 years (14–64 yo), reflecting the fact that a large part of pectus excavatum are not corrected in childhood. Psychological difficulties often develop in adolescence or adulthood (sometimes late adulthood), motivating consultations. Such patients are frequently seen as adults and often request surgery that is rapid, not disabling, and not associated with prolonged effects on work and sport.

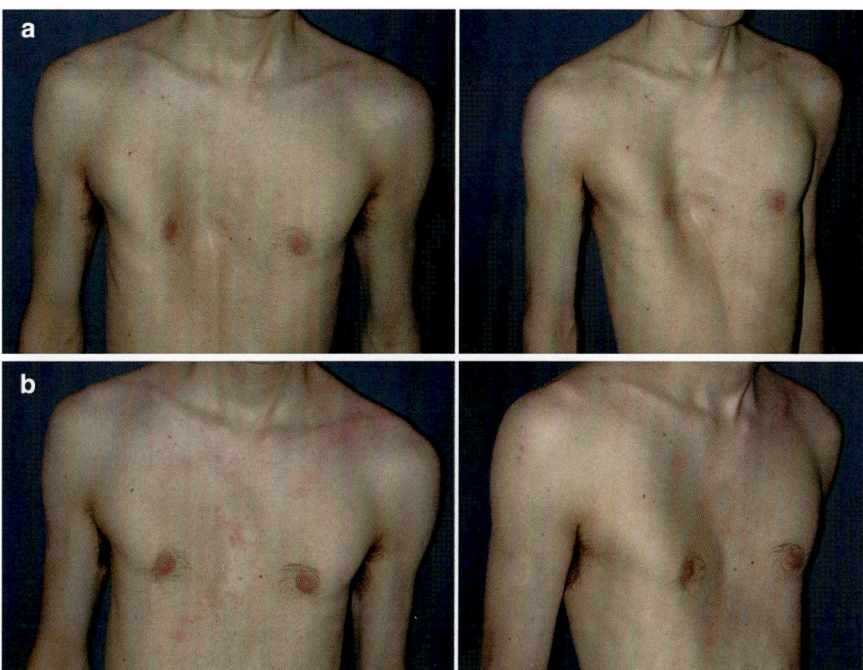

Fig. 3.14 Pectus excavatum type 3 in a man: (**a**) before, (**b**) 1 year later

Our initial procedure (external plaster moulding) yielded good results because of a submuscular position, but (sometimes) barely detectable imperfections in contour or volume were evident. This was attributable to the interposition of soft tissues such as breasts in females or well-developed muscles in males in an effort to hide the deformation, sometimes asymmetrically. CAD with 3D reconstruction renders implant's design perfect; the thoracic deformation, especially deep and asymmetric, is minutely charted (Fig. 3.12). The results on athletic men (Fig. 3.13) and asymmetric women (Fig. 3.11) are especially demonstrative.

Custom-made silicone implants are now perfectly made in 3D conception and manufacturing; more and more surgeons of any specialty (plastic, thoracic, paediatric) are convinced by these implants, although very few relevant articles have appeared, with relatively small patient numbers.

Seroma was detected clinically in every case. In our series, the pectoralis major bilateral medial section and submuscular undermining explain the quasi-constant seroma; unlike the cited authors, we never placed the implants subcutaneously. In the first years, we used suction drain. Nonetheless, after removing the drain, seroma occurs frequently, so we chose to stop their use. The seroma requires three punctures [2–5] during the first post-operative month but never becomes chronic.

No periprosthetic capsular contracture formed around the implants in the long term. Unlike breast implants filled with soft silicone gel, the silicone elastomer implants are semi-rigid, and we thus assume that they neither retract nor contract. In

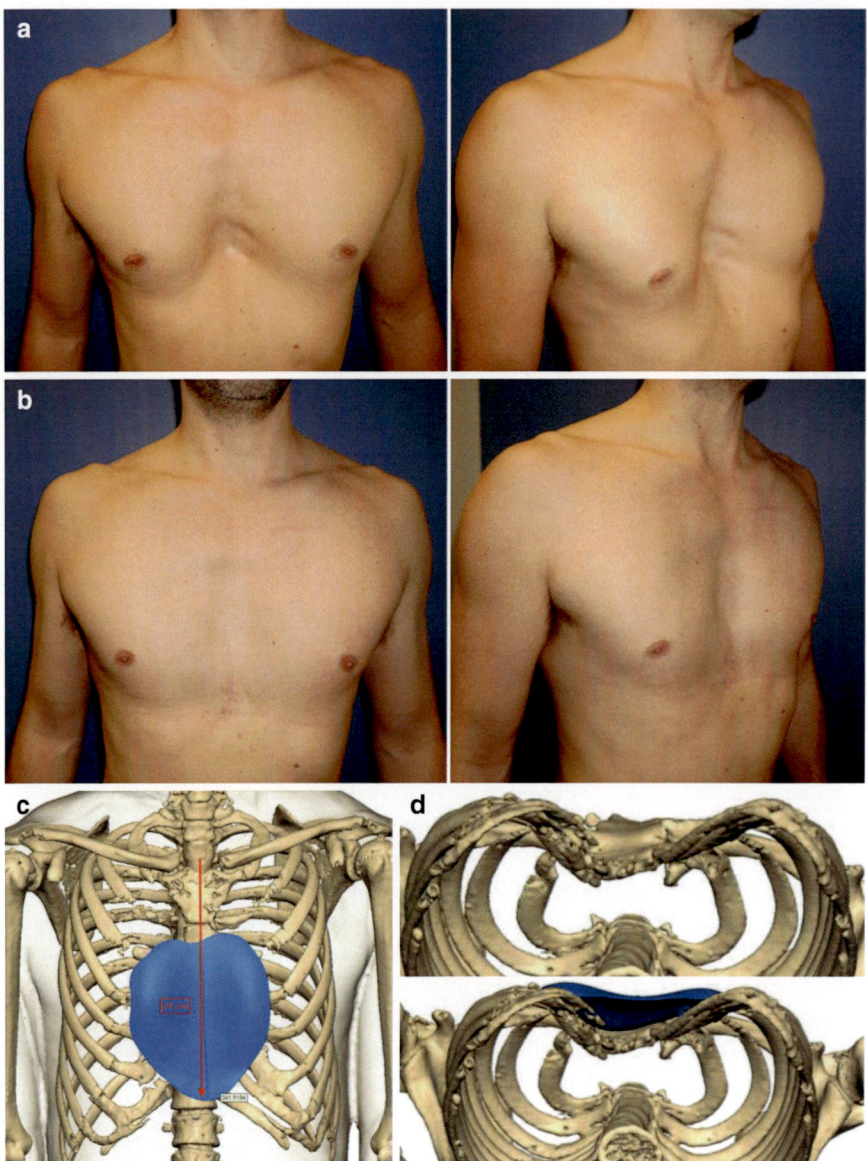

Fig. 3.15 Pectus excavatum type 1 in an athletic man: (**a**) before, (**b**) 1 year later, (**c**) CAD front face, (**d**) CAD supine

the absence of fracture, rupture, or degradation, the elastomer silicone implant is retained for life.

Although psychological and cosmetic considerations remain the main indications for pectus excavatum repair, few studies have explored patient satisfaction and the aesthetic results and do not include any work involving CAD to create silicone implants.

In terms of cosmetic assessment, both the patients and the surgeons consider that the outcomes are good to excellent, being significantly better in the CAD than the first plaster group. In terms of satisfaction, 80% of patients reconstructed via CAD were satisfied or very satisfied (scores 4 and 5), reflecting principally the cosmetic results. No specific scale evaluating the effect of pectus excavatum on QOL exists, and we thus employed the MOS-SF36, one of the most widely used and internationally validated scales. Significant improvements in social and emotional functioning were evident, especially in the CAD group; the patients had functioned rather poorly prior to surgery. Other parameters including "general and mental health" and "role physical" also improved, but the between-group differences were not significant.

The reported pain associated with implant placement was highlighted on the MOS-SF36 ("bodily pain"). We have not encountered this complaint before, and the literature is silent on the topic. Patients reported that they could feel the prostheses during certain intense sporting activities, as may also be the case for breast implants, for example. We believe that the medium- and long-term pain associated with remodelling thoracic surgery are greatly underestimated or not evaluated in various

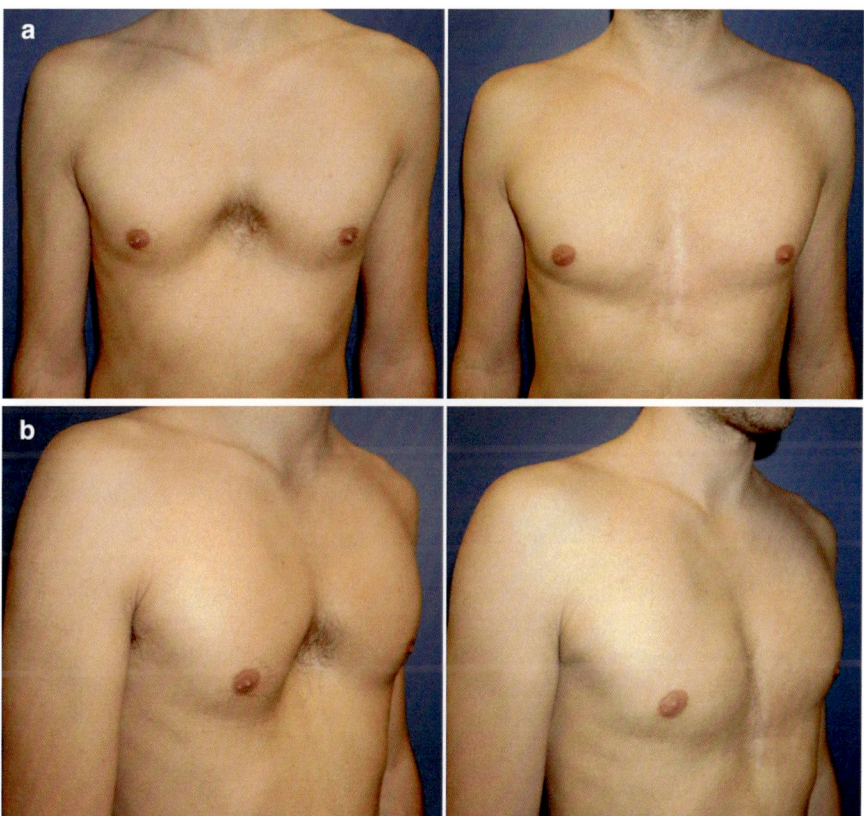

Fig. 3.16 Pectus arcuatum type 4 in a male: (**a**) before, (**b**) 1 year later, (**c**) CAD front face, (**d**) CAD supine

Fig. 3.16 (continued)

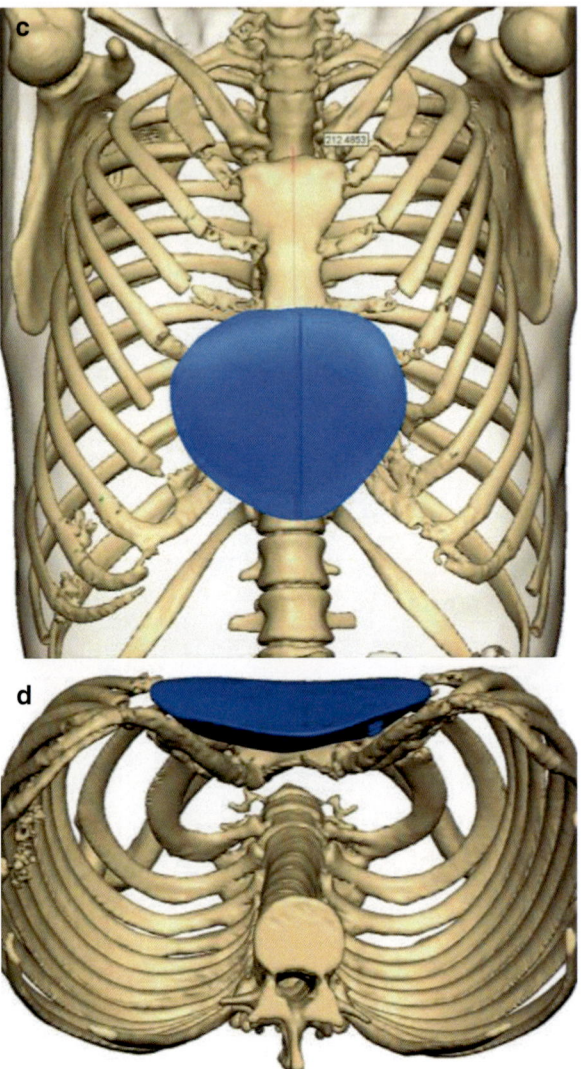

publications, and it is thus difficult to compare such patients with those of our series. It should also be noted that, in retrospective studies, pain reports are often unreliable. The feel of the prosthesis during physical effort was described more as discomfort than pain. Only two patients have ever requested the removal of prosthesis. For all other cases, the discomfort and sport restriction are very short and low compared with the pain induced by the two orthopaedic procedures of the modified Ravitch and Nuss.

To the best of our knowledge, this is the largest series of pectus excavatum corrections using custom-made silicone implants with the help of CAD to be reported in the literature. Also, we present a long-term follow-up, showing stability of the implants and the results.

All of our demographic and surgical data were collected prospectively, but the cosmetic self-evaluation and QOL assessment were retrospective in nature, with the limitations inherent to retrospectivity.

3.5   Conclusions

We managed pectus excavatum patients on a strictly cosmetic basis after control of respiratory and cardiac function. Custom-made implants designed using 3D CT data afforded good-to-excellent cosmetic results in most patients, who were generally satisfied and enjoyed an improved QOL. The inevitable seroma poses few risks.

Both remodelling thoracic surgeries and silicone implants correct pectus excavatum, affording significant cosmetic improvements with good patient satisfaction and QOL improvement. So, we suggest that the simplest and less invasive procedure should be preferred; the risk of complications is low and morbidity much reduced. The benefit-risk report is very low, compared with other procedures cited. The medico-economic cost is far lower too: only one procedure, quick recovery, lower cost of material, no recurrences or possible heavy complications.

References

1. Creswick HA, Stacey MW, Kelly RE, Gustin T, Nuss D, Harvey H, et al. Family study of the inheritance of pectus excavatum. J Pediatr Surg. 2006;41(10):1699–703.
2. Krasopoulos G, Goldstraw P. Minimally invasive repair of pectus excavatum deformity. Eur J Cardiothorac Surg. 2011;39(2):149–58.
3. Nuss D, Kelly RE. Minimally invasive surgical correction of chest wall deformities in children (nuss procedure). Adv Pediatr. 2008;55(1):395–410.
4. Lawson ML, Cash TF, Akers R, Vasser E, Burke B, Tabangin M, et al. A pilot study of the impact of surgical repair on disease-specific quality of life among patients with pectus excavatum. J Pediatr Surg. 2003;38(6):916–8.
5. Hong J-Y, Suh S-W, Park H-J, Kim Y-H, Park J-H, Park S-Y. Correlations of adolescent idiopathic scoliosis and pectus excavatum. J Pediatr Orthop. 2011;31(8):870–4.
6. Lomholt JJ, Jacobsen EB, Thastum M, Pilegaard H. A prospective study on quality of life in youths after pectus excavatum correction. Ann Cardiothorac Surg. 2016;5(5):456–65.
7. Steinmann C, Krille S, Mueller A, Weber P, Reingruber B, Martin A. Pectus excavatum and pectus carinatum patients suffer from lower quality of life and impaired body image: a control group comparison of psychological characteristics prior to surgical correction. Eur J Cardiothorac Surg. 2011;40(5):1138–45.
8. Ji Y, Liu W, Chen S, Xu B, Tang Y, Wang X, et al. Assessment of psychosocial functioning and its risk factors in children with pectus excavatum. Health Qual Life Outcomes. 2011;9:28.
9. Malek MH, Berger DE, Housh TJ, Marelich WD, Coburn JW, Beck TW. Cardiovascular function following surgical repair of pectus excavatum: a metaanalysis. Chest. 2006;130(2):506–16.
10. Malek MH, Berger DE, Marelich WD, Coburn JW, Beck TW, Housh TJ. Pulmonary function following surgical repair of pectus excavatum: a meta-analysis. Eur J Cardiothorac Surg. 2006;30(4):637–43.
11. Guntheroth WG, Spiers PS. Cardiac function before and after surgery for pectus excavatum. Am J Cardiol. 2007;99(12):1762–4.

12. Fonkalsrud EW, Dunn JCY, Atkinson JB. Repair of pectus excavatum deformities: 30 years of experience with 375 patients. Ann Surg. 2000;231(3):443–8.
13. Del Frari B, Schwabegger AH. Clinical results and patient satisfaction after pectus excavatum repair using the MIRPE and MOVARPE technique in adults: 10-year experience. Plast Reconstr Surg. 2013;132(6):1591–602.
14. Kelly RE, Goretsky MJ, Obermeyer R, Kuhn MA, Redlinger R, Haney TS, et al. Twenty-one years of experience with minimally invasive repair of pectus excavatum by the Nuss procedure in 1215 patients. Ann Surg. 2010;252(6):1072–81.
15. Pilegaard HK. Nuss technique in pectus excavatum: a mono-institutional experience. J Thorac Dis. 2015;7(Suppl 2):S172–6.
16. Schwabegger AH, Del Frari B, Pierer G. Aesthetic improvement of the female breast in funnel chest deformity by surgical repair of the thoracic wall: indication or lifestyle surgery? Plast Reconstr Surg. 2012;130(2):245e.
17. Ho Quoc C, Delaporte T, Meruta A, La Marca S, Toussoun G, Delay E. Breast asymmetry and pectus excavatum improvement with fat grafting. Aesthet Surg J. 2013;33(6):822–9.
18. Chavoin JP, Dahan M, Grolleau JL, Soubirac L, Wagner A, Foucras L, et al. Funnel chest: filling technique with deep custom made implant. Ann Chir Plast Esthet. 2003;48(2):67–76.
19. Andre A, Bozonnet E, Dahan M, Chavoin JP. Correction chirurgicale du pectus excavatum par prothèse pariétale en silicone sur mesure. chapitre 11. In: JP. Chavoin, editor. Chirurgie plastique et reconstructrice des parois et des confins, Rapport 2009. SOFCPRE (Société Française de chirurgie Plastique Reconstructrice et esthétique). Paris: Elsevier-Masson; 2009. p. 138–57.
20. Chavoin J-P, Grolleau J-L, Moreno B, Brunello J, André A, Dahan M, et al. Correction of pectus excavatum by custom-made silicone implants: contribution of computer-aided design reconstruction. a 20-year experience and 401 cases. Plast Reconstr Surg. 2016;137(5):860e–71e.
21. Chin EF, Adler RH. The surgical treatment of pectus excavatum (funnel chest). Br Med J. 1954;1(4870):1064–6.
22. Murray J. Correction of pectus excavatum by synthetic subcutaneous implant. American Society of Plastic and Reconstructive Surgery; 1965.
23. Toty L, Hertzog P, Rotten D. Correction plastique du pectus excavatum par une prothèse en silastic préparée extemporanément. Rev Fr Mal Resp. 1973;11:1153–9.
24. Marks M, Argenta L, Lee D. Silicone implant correction of pectus excavatum: indications and refinement in technique. Plast Reconstr Surg. 1984:74, 52–8.
25. Johnson PE. Refining silicone implant correction of pectus excavatum through computed tomography. Plast Reconstr Surg. 1996;97(2):445.
26. Mendelson B, Masson JK. Silicone implants for contour deformities of the trunk. Plast Reconstr Surg. 1977;59(4):538–44.
27. Johan Nordquist MJ, Svensson H. Silastic implant for reconstruction of pectus excavatum: an update. Scand J Plast Reconstr Surg Hand Surg. 2001;35(1):65–9.
28. Wechselberger G, Öhlbauer M, Haslinger J, Schoeller T, Bauer T, Piza-Katzer H. Silicone implant correction of pectus excavatum. Ann Plast Surg. 2001;47(5):489–93.
29. Margulis A, Sela M, Neuman R, Buller-Sharon A. Reconstruction of pectus excavatum with silicone implants. J Plast Reconstr Aesthet Surg. 2006;59(10):1082–6.
30. Horch RE, Stoelben E, Carbon R, Sultan AA, Bach AD, Kneser U. Pectus excavatum breast and chest deformity: indications for aesthetic plastic surgery versus thoracic surgery in a multicenter experience. Aesthetic Plast Surg. 2006;30(4):403–11.
31. Poupon M, Duteille F, Casanova D, Caye N, Magalon G, Pannier M. [Pectus excavatum: what treatment in plastic surgery? About 10 cases]. Ann Chir Plast Esthet. 2008;53(3):246–54.
32. Snel BJ, Spronk CA, Werker PMN, van der Lei B. Pectus excavatum reconstruction with silicone implants: long-term results and a review of the english-language literature. Ann Plast Surg. 2009;62(2):205–9.
33. Einsiedel E, Clausner A. Funnel chest. Psychological and psychosomatic aspects in children, youngsters, and young adults - ProQuest. J Card Surg. 1999;40:733–6.
34. Frantz FW. Indications and guidelines for pectus excavatum repair. Curr Opin Pediatr. 2011;23(4):486–91.

35. Kim HK, Shim JH, Choi KS, Choi YH. The quality of life after bar removal in patients after the nuss procedure for pectus excavatum. World J Surg. 2011;35(7):1656–61.
36. Kelly RE, Cash TF, Shamberger RC, Mitchell KK, Mellins RB, Lawson ML, et al. Surgical repair of pectus excavatum markedly improves body image and perceived ability for physical activity: multicenter study. Pediatrics. 2008;122(6):1218–22.
37. Schier F, Bahr M, Klobe E. The vacuum chest wall lifter: an innovative, nonsurgical addition to the management of pectus excavatum. J Pediatr Surg. 2005;40(3):496–500.
38. Haecker F-M, Sesia S. Non-surgical treatment of pectus excavatum. J Visc Surg. 2016;2:63.
39. Pereira LH, Sterodimas A. Free fat transplantation for the aesthetic correction of mild pectus excavatum. Aesthetic Plast Surg. 2008;32(2):393–6.

Poland Syndrome Remodeling by CAD Silicone Custom-Made Implants

4

Jean-Pierre Chavoin, Mohcine Taizou, Benjamin Moreno, Jean-Louis Grolleau, and Benoit Chaput

4.1   Introduction

Poland syndrome is associated with varying degrees of thoracic abnormalities and malformations of the upper limbs. The pathognomonic anomaly is agenesis of the sternocostal fibers of the pectoralis major [1]. Breast asymmetry occurs frequently in women [2] but the rate of hand malformations varies widely [3]. Poland syndrome is a rare malformation, as the incidence is estimated at only 1 per 30,000 births [4]. There appears to be a male predominance (3:1), and the majority of studies attest to lateralization of Poland syndrome on the right side. The etiology of the syndrome remains unknown but a vascular origin, as supported by Bavinck and Weaver [5], could explain the existence of associated syndromes (pectus, tuberous breasts).

The extent of breast and chest-wall deformities varies widely in Poland syndrome. This is due to the variable degree of tissue's atrophy not only the muscular plane, but also the chest bone, cutaneous and sub-cutaneous planes (with the breast

Electronic Supplementary Material The online version of this chapter (https://doi. org/10.1007/978-3-030-05108-2_4) contains supplementary material, which is available to authorized users.

J.-P. Chavoin (✉) · M. Taizou · J.-L. Grolleau · B. Chaput
Plastic Surgery Department, Rangueil Hospital, Toulouse University Hospital, Toulouse, France
e-mail: jean-pierre.chavoin@orange.fr; mohcine.taizou@orange.fr; grolleau.jl@chu-toulouse.fr; chaput.b@chu-toulouse.fr

B. Moreno
AnatomikModeling, 19 Rue Jean Mermoz, Toulouse, France
e-mail: bmoreno@anatomikmodeling.com

© Springer Nature Switzerland AG 2019
J.-P. Chavoin (ed.), *Pectus Excavatum and Poland Syndrome Surgery*,
https://doi.org/10.1007/978-3-030-05108-2_4

in women). Surgeons must master several techniques to treat all of these atrophies. Thus, several authors have proposed decision algorithms, based on their experience (often short and with mild results), but implementation is sometimes difficult [2, 6–8]. However, a customized technique perfectly suited to the malformation can be used for the majority of patients. Thus, in 2007, we developed an innovative computer-aided design (CAD) procedure for thoracic implant reconstruction of patients with Poland syndrome using a thin-section scanner [9, 10]. This minimally invasive procedure consists in placing permanent, custom-made silicone elastomer implants to fill defects due to muscular agenesis and, sometimes, the associated thoracic atrophies.

In our experience, we objectively evaluated the esthetic improvement and quality of life (QoL) of Poland syndrome patients who underwent reconstruction with three-dimensional (3D) CAD custom-made implants. We also have compared the quality of the reconstruction in men and women, for whom reconstruction imperatives often differ. Patient demographics and symptoms are discussed, and the surgical technique is described.

4.2   Patients and Methods

Since 1993, we have treated 138 patients for Poland syndrome thoracic malformations in our plastic and reconstructive surgery unit (Toulouse, Rangueil, France). All available thoracic reconstruction techniques are explained to the patients both orally and with information documents. From 1993 to 2007, we used plaster molds of the thorax to prepare silicone implants ($n = 15$). Since 2007, we have used preoperative 3D volume-rendered computed tomography scans to design implants for 76 patients.

All patients are adults, we use the classification of Foucras et al., described by our team in 2003 [2], and added the type IV classification, corresponding to previously operated-in patients [2]. We recontacted by telephone, or arranged an in-person consultation, with patients who had undergone reconstruction with 3D CAD silicone implants ($n = 68$). Patient satisfaction is evaluated retrospectively using standardized questionnaires and QoL was assessed using the MOS-SF36 questionnaire.

4.2.1   Manufacture of Custom Implants via Computer-Aided Design

As for pectus excavatum, three steps are required to prepare the implants (as described in Chap. 2). First, a computed tomography (CT) scan is obtained, with 1–1.2 mm slice thickness, during which *the patients keep their arms along the body*: it is essential to avoid a muscle extension on the normal side which will be used and copied for digital reconstruction of the atrophied side. A computer scientist reconstructs the missing space between the deep plane, termed the "surgical plane" (ribcage, intercostal spaces) and the superficial plane, termed the "anatomical plane," to virtually correct asymmetry due to muscle and sometimes chest asymmetry, and enhance breast positioning in women. AnatomikModeling (Toulouse, France) prepares the 3D CAD digital image model of the implant.

Implant prototypes are manufactured from the 3D models using a 3D computerized numerical control milling machine. Each implant is made based on the molding and casting, using a silicone elastomer (Nusil). The implant is semi-rigid, highly flexible, tear resistant, and gas sterilized. Such implants can be retained for the duration of the patient's life when the result is good.

4.2.2   Surgical Technique and Follow-up

General anesthesia with intubation or laryngeal mask is applied to all patients in the supine position, with the arms first along the thorax. We routinely prescribe an intraoperative prophylactic antibiotic (2 g of intravenous cefazolin injected at the start the surgery).

Before decontamination, the lower point is exactly positioned using a computerized marker (distance between the inter-clavicular sternal fork and the caudal margin of the implant) (Fig. 4.1).

Then, the prototype is put on the thorax, arms along the body to ensure optimal positioning. We trace the perimeter of the implant, thereby defining the limits of implant's position (Fig. 4.2).

Afterwards, the arm is positioned in abduction to allow an axillary approach in a lazy S shape 8 cm long (Fig. 4.3).

Fig. 4.1 Implant's lower pole is exactly positioned using a computerized marker

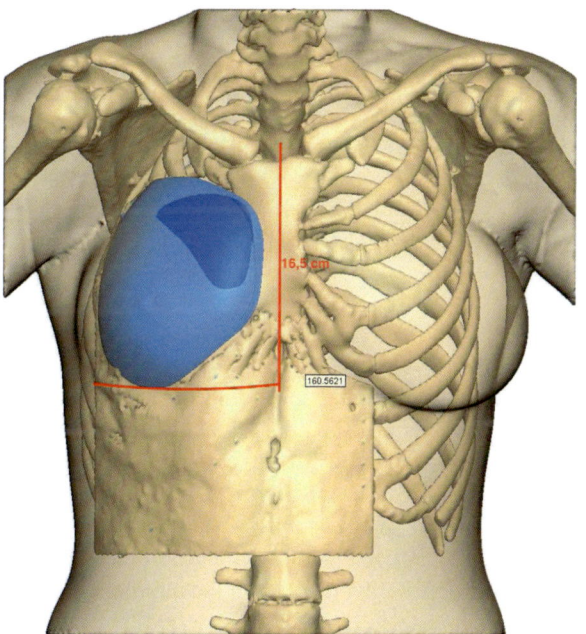

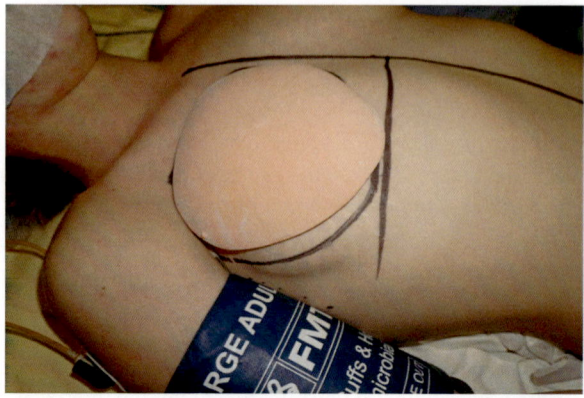

Fig. 4.2 Perimeter of the implant is traced around the prototype in good position, arm along the body

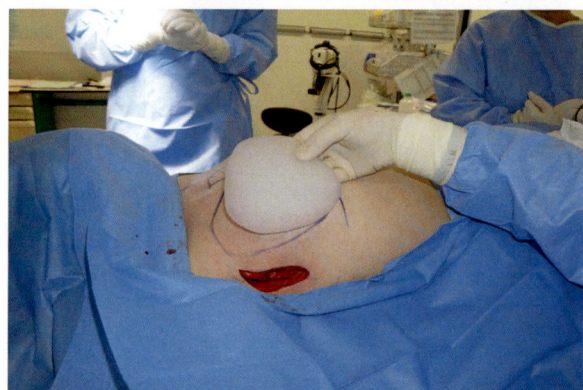

Fig. 4.3 Axillary approach in a lazy S shape of 8 cm length seen just before implantation

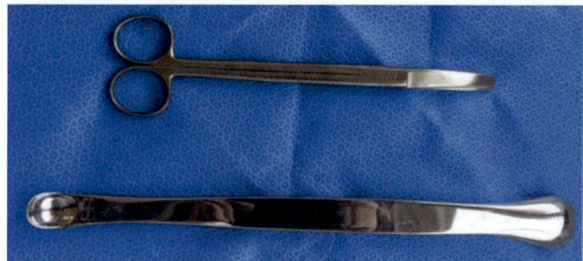

Fig. 4.4 Two instruments can be used: long curved Mayo scissors and Lambotte rugina

Section is done to the level of the deep thoracic plane, taking account of the serratus pedicle located behind. Dissection of the pre-costal space is done first with scissors, and then by fingers, to complete the sub-cutaneous undermining.

In cases of a resistant fibrous septum, long curved Mayo scissors or Lambotte rugina are used (Fig. 4.4). Hemostasis is controlled but the procedure was often not hemorrhagic. Patients with Poland syndrome are likely to have embryological atrophy of the perforating pedicles of the internal mammary. The soft elastomer implant is folded in on itself and easily inserted through the axillary path (Fig. 4.5). The

Fig. 4.5 The soft elastomer implant can be folded in on itself and easily inserted through the axillary path

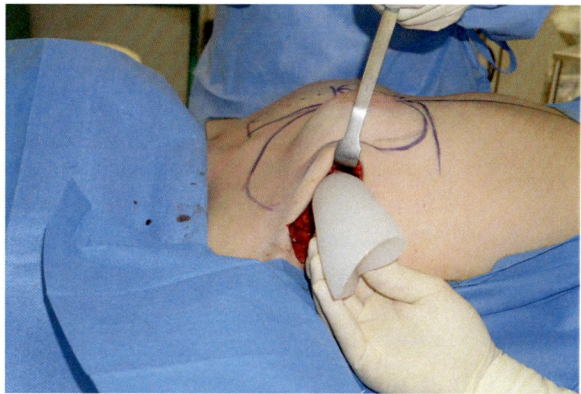

Fig. 4.6 Correct orientation of the implant is verified by an axillary mark (button)

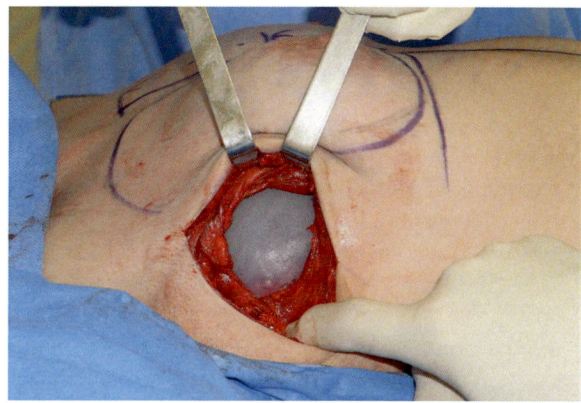

implant redeploys spontaneously in the sub-cutaneous pocket. The semi-rigid consistency of the implant facilitates folding and easy insertion but it is also undeformable. Correct orientation of the implant is verified laterally by an axillary mark (button) (Fig. 4.6) and by a medial edge line added during manufacture. Closure is done in two planes, using resorbable wires and without any drainage. Then, we put a dressing then a mildly compressive bandage with polyurethane (Microfoam Ethicon®) for 2 days.

After hospitalization the patient has to keep a light bra (Romeo type Medical Z®) for 15 days.

The dressing is not changed during the first week. Most patients return to work after 2 weeks. The bra is kept on for 15 days. Sports activities are stopped for 2 months.

4.3   Results

The demographic data and operative characteristics of the 138 patients: sex ratio 6 men for 4 women; mean age, 26 years; range: 9–40 years. The mean number of interventions was 1.82 (range: 1–6) and type I malformation was the most common.

The patients benefited from the application of different surgical procedures, including CAD custom-made silicone implants (52.7%), lipofilling (42.6%), mammary prostheses (24.8%), custom-made silicone implants by plaster molds (11.6%), latissimus dorsi flap (3.1%), and thoracic remodeling surgery (0.7%).

Here, we were mainly interested in reconstructions using 3D CAD implants. We treated 75 patients consecutively with the 3D CAD silicone implant during the period 2007–2017. The mean operative time was 49 min (range: 40–78 min), and the mean length of hospital stay was 4.2 days (range: 2–8 days).

Even if the symmetry is not always strictly perfect, and the consistency too firm compared to a true muscle, these silicone elastomer implants give often good results on men even athletics (Fig. 4.7) very rarely bilateral (Fig. 4.8). For women, it can be with the chest implant only to improve a pure chest asymmetry (Fig. 4.9). Nine women (41%) received a breast implant, and this was always performed a second time to allow the implant pocket of the CAD prosthesis to form. We take care not to reopen the anterior fibrous capsule of the first implant by careful placement of the breast prosthesis to avoid sliding and implant's displacement. Therefore, if the asymmetry is due to muscle atrophy but also a breast unilateral hypotrophy, two procedures will be done in at least 6 months interval (Fig. 4.10): first chest implant, then breast implant always separated by the fibrous capsule of the previous one.

A complementary lipofilling procedure was carried out as a second step in 20.6% of the patients to optimize the results.

Two postoperative hematomas (1.6%) that required re-intervention were recorded as complications. We experienced two infections following lipofilling procedures and removal was required in three cases of long-term prosthetic exposure. The axillary location of the scar seemed to prevent wound dehiscence. Two patients requested removal of their prosthesis, one due to pain and the other due to psychological difficulty in accepting the presence of a foreign body. Peri-prosthetic seromas were found in 20.5% of cases, and these required puncture before resolving spontaneously. The absence of muscle section tended to result in seroma disappearance in our most recent cases. No implant exhibited capsular contracture, and we noticed no rupture or displacement of the implant.

Concerning global patient satisfaction, about 77% of the women and >80% of the men were "satisfied" or "very satisfied" (scores of 4 and 5, respectively) with their reconstruction, without significant difference between the two sexes.

We have significant improvements in both social and emotional aspects. Pain ("body pain") associated with the prosthesis was significant in both groups. All patients described discomfort during intense sporting activities, but without pain that was quantifiable on a visual analog scale. Ultimately, "general health" tends to be improved in both the men and women.

4.4   Discussion

Poland syndrome remains a complex malformed entity with various clinical presentations. Many techniques have been proposed to correct the malformations, which often lead to acceptable but poor results. The latissimus dorsi flap remains for some

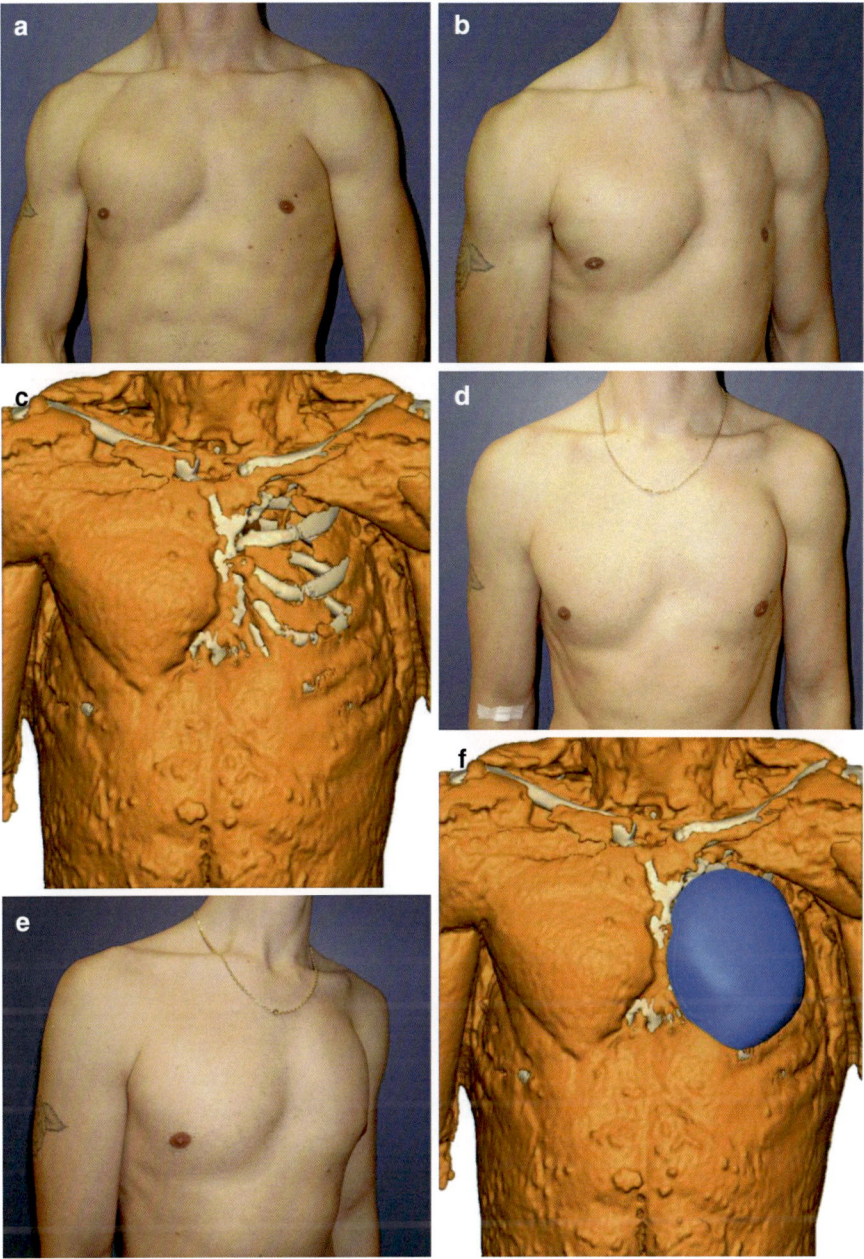

Fig. 4.7 Poland syndrome type 2 on an athletic man before (**a**, **b**), 1 year after (**d**, **e**); CAD with muscles segmentation (**c**) and implant's image front face (**f**)

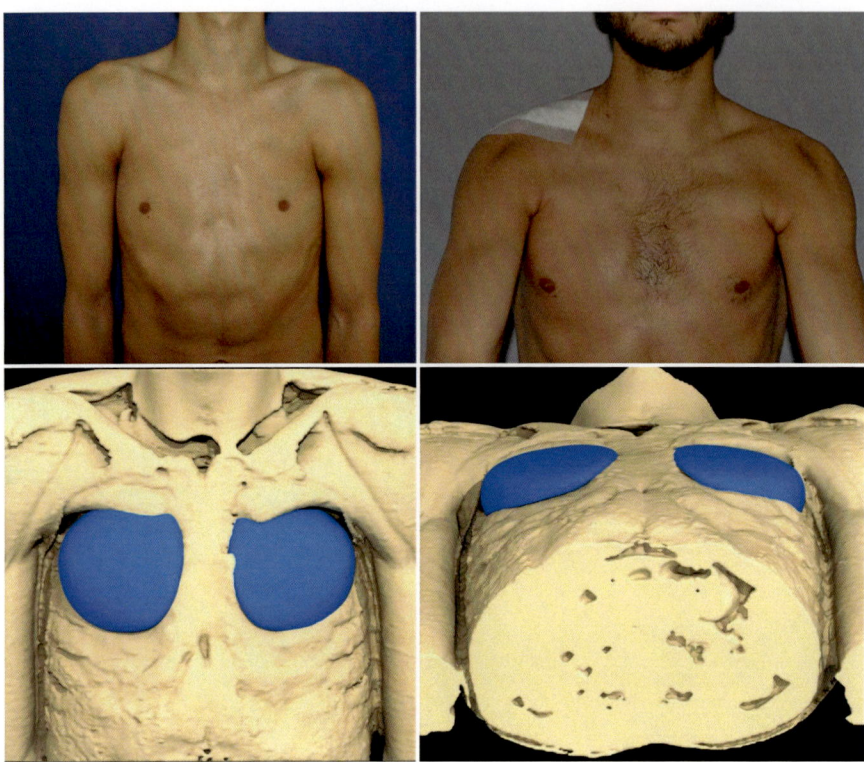

Fig. 4.8 A very rare bilateral Poland syndrome before and 1 year after reconstruction with two implants

the gold standard [8, 11, 12] but we nevermore use it since 24 years: our last case has been recently treated with an implant (Fig. 4.11). Moreover, tissue expansion [2], transverse rectus abdominis flap [13], an omentum flap [8, 14], and thoracic remodeling surgery [15], alone or in combination, are no more to be used. The use of perforator flaps has also been described, such as the free deep inferior epigastric perforator flap [16] or pedicled thoracodorsal artery perforator flap [17]. Nonetheless, some of these procedures have high morbidity, and case series are limited.

Fat transfer techniques are highly assistive in minor malformation, resulting in significant improvement in patients, but in most deformations the limits of this treatment are quickly exceeded [18]. Moreover, lipofilling has been used widely to allow additional corrective procedures, or to prepare the tissue before placing a prosthesis and, thus improve atrophy of the chest wall. We have been reluctant to practice this procedure near the mammary gland but it seems to be well established and the neoplastic risk is very low [19–21] until now.

Even in the presence of a rib or thoracic malformation, or an associated pectus excavatum, there is no evidence of cardiac or respiratory functional consequences of the thoracic malformations that occur in patients with Poland syndrome.

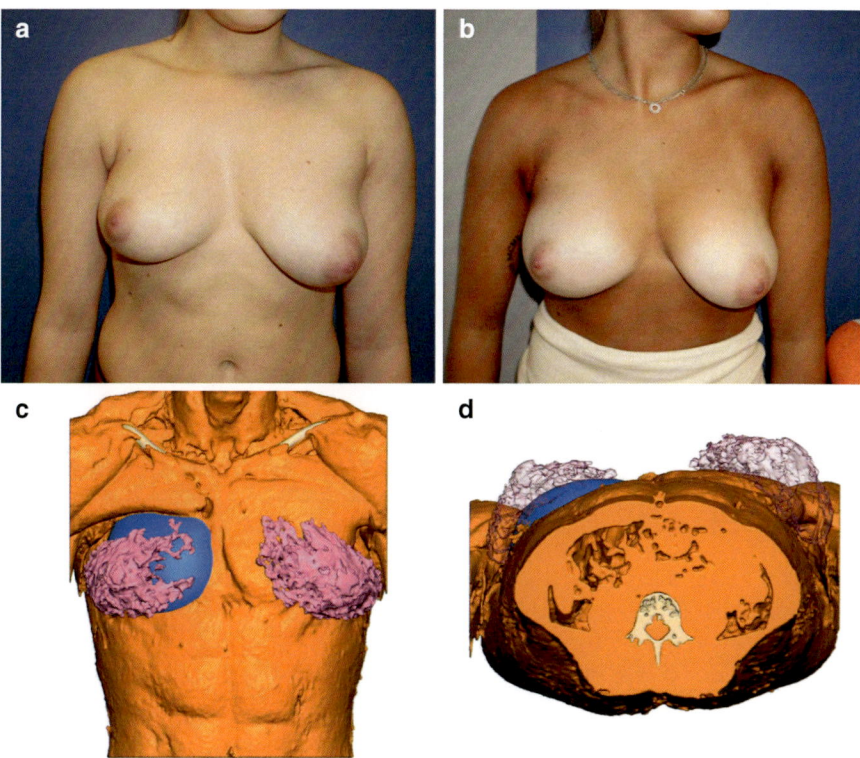

Fig. 4.9 Poland's type 1 on a woman with pure chest asymmetry: before (**a**) and 1 year (**b**) after CAD implant's 3D reconstruction front face (**c**) and supine position (**d**)

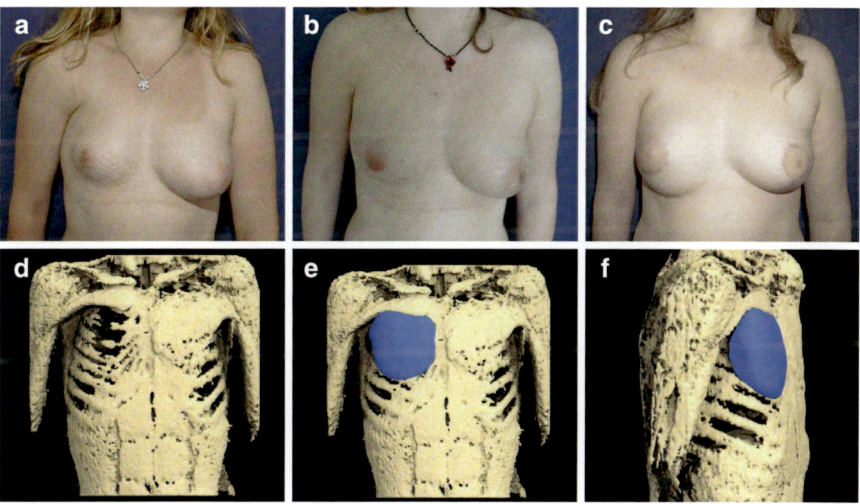

Fig. 4.10 Poland's type 2 on a woman with an ipsilateral breast hypotrophy is reconstructed in two procedures separated with 1-year interval (**a–c**) with 3D procedure (**d–f**)

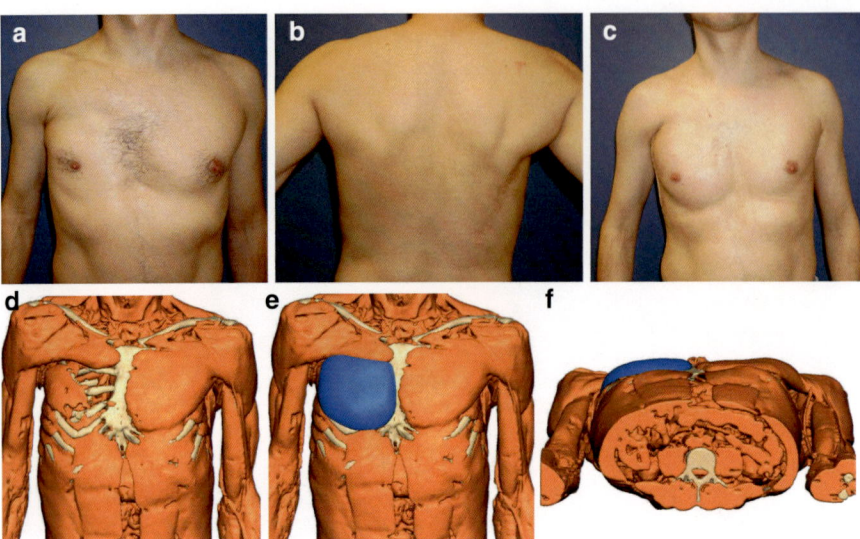

Fig. 4.11 Failure of a personal latissimus dorsi flap 25 years after (**a**), sequela on the back (**b**), result after 3 months (**c**) and CAD implant's 3D reconstruction front face and supine position (**d–f**)

It is necessary to be aware that an esthetic result and perfect symmetry are extremely difficult to obtain in patients with Poland syndrome; this must be relayed to the patient from the outset. The technical and surgical requirements for reconstruction differ between men and women, and it seems that reconstruction with CAD implants makes it possible to obtain satisfactory results in both sexes. Nevertheless, women often require implantation of a breast prosthesis, as in 41% of the cases in our series showing frequent mammary hypoplasia.

Our initial implant preparation technique using an external plaster mold yielded good results, but barely detectable imperfections in terms of contour or volume were occasionally evident. This was attributable to the interposition of soft tissues, such as breasts in females or well-developed muscles in males, in an effort to camouflage the deformation, with occasionally asymmetric results. These tissues varied in thickness and location, which compromised the plaster molding. In addition, the implant was more likely to be visible or detectable by touch when the skin was thin but 3D CAD allowed for rendering of a more optimized prosthetic design. With 3D CAD, prosthesis contours were softened, and the volume was always underestimated by 15–20% to avoid the maximum contour when the skin was thin.

We experienced only two hematomas and two infections, secondary to lipofilling, as complications. The hematomas required re-operations, and the infections necessitated removal of the prosthesis and cessation of antibiotic treatment. Seromas formed in 20.5% of cases during the early postoperative period and were the most frequently observed minor complications. These seromas were treated with one or two aspirations during the first postoperative month but always resorbed. No patient developed a residual seroma after 3 months. Patients should be told to expect a seroma, and aspiration should be done by a surgeon to avoid any risk of infection. No peri-prosthetic capsular contracture is formed around the implants in the long term. Unlike breast implants filled with soft silicone gel, silicone elastomer implants are semi-rigid; thus, we assumed that they would neither retract nor contract. In the absence of a fracture, rupture, or degradation, the prosthesis is retained for the duration of the patient's life.

Since 2007, we have completely abandoned other procedures, such as the latissimus dorsi approach, which over time produces atrophy and leaving behind a dorsal sequelae (Fig. 4.7) but also isolated mammary prostheses that did not respond to the actual deformation. Finally, we have never obtained sufficient and symmetrical results using the lipofilling procedure alone, as reported by the Delay team [22]; this often requires three to five procedures, some times more. The other negative aspect of lipofilling for men is that they are often young, thin, and muscular patients, and thus it is difficult to find an adipose tissue donor site.

This technique is minimally invasive, rapid, and associated with very low morbidity. Asymmetries >200 mL can be corrected during a single operation with very good accuracy, by compensating for the loss of muscle volume, and leave a discrete axillary scar. Nevertheless, custom-made silicone implants are complex to model and expensive, so few surgeons employ such prostheses. Very few relevant articles have appeared regarding these implants, and those that have used a relatively small number of patients. In 1991, Marks presented a series of eight patients with customized silicone implants covered directly by the latissimus dorsi and achieved satisfactory results in 50% of cases [7]. In 2003, Foucras, in our team, published a series of 10 patients with mixed results because the implants were prepared using plaster molds [2]. Perignon et al., in 2009, reported a very esthetic reconstruction using a plaster mold in a male patient [22]. The only minor complication was a 100-cm^3 seroma requiring puncture. In 2015, Majdak considered custom-made silicone implants very useful for moderate deformations [6]. However, none of these authors employed CAD using 3D CT data.

The recent study of Baldelli et al. highlights that patient should be operated on during the period of growth to allow for proper body image stabilization and improved QoL. With our technique, it is possible to operate on patients relatively early, i.e., just after puberty. If the prosthesis becomes too small, it is always possible to redo it or to perform secondary lipofilling. The mean patient age in our series was 26 years, reflecting that a large proportion of patients are uncorrected during childhood. Psychological difficulties often develop in adolescence or adulthood, motivating consultations. Such patients are frequently seen for the first time as adults, and often request surgery that is rapid, and not disabling or associated with prolonged effects on work or sports activities. Although psychological and cosmetic considerations remain the main indications for treating Poland syndrome, few studies have explored patient satisfaction and esthetic results, and none include any work done involving CAD to create silicone implants. In the present study, both men and women considered that the outcomes of the CAD implants were good to excellent. In terms of overall satisfaction, 76.9% of women and >80% of men rated that they were "satisfied" or "very satisfied," demonstrating that this technique gives good results in both sexes.

This result demonstrates that reconstruction improved patient body image [10, 23].

Pain reports are often unreliable in retrospective studies. The experience of the prosthesis during physical effort was described more as discomfort than pain and only one patient requested removal of the prosthesis for pain-related reasons.

To the best of our knowledge, this is the largest reported series of Poland syndrome corrections using CAD custom silicone implants. We also present long-term follow-up data, showing the stability of the implants and outcomes.

4.5   Conclusions

We managed patients with Poland syndrome on a strictly cosmetic basis. Custom implants designed using 3D CT data afforded good-to-excellent cosmetic results in most patients, who were generally satisfied and enjoyed both in social and emotional terms. This procedure allows for the management of the majority of defects alone or with secondary breast implant or lipofilling to enhance the result.

References

1. Poland A. Deficiency of the pectoral muscles. Guys Hosp Rep. 1841;6:191–3.
2. Foucras L, Grolleau-Raoux JL, Chavoin JP. [Poland's syndrome: clinic series and thoraco-mammary reconstruction. Report of 27 cases]. Ann Chir Plast Esthet. 2003;48(2):54–66.
3. Foucras L, Grolleau JL, Chavoin JP. [Poland'syndrome and hand's malformations: about a clinic series of 37 patients]. Ann Chir Plast Esthet. 2005;50(2):138–45 (French).
4. McGillivray BC, Lowry RB. Poland syndrome in British Columbia: incidence and reproductive experience of affected persons. Am J Med Genet. 1977;1:65–74.
5. Bavinck JN, Weaver DD. Subclavian artery supply disruption sequence: hypothesis of a vascular etiology for Poland, Klippel-Feil and Moebius anomalies. Am J Med Genet. 1986;23:903–18.
6. Majdak-Paredes EJ, Shafighi M, Fatah F. Integrated algorithm for reconstruction of complex forms of Poland syndrome: 20-year outcomes. J Plast Reconstr Aesthet Surg. 2015;68(10):1386–94.
7. Baldelli I, Santi P, Dova L, Cardoni G, Ciliberti R, Franchelli S, Merlo DF, Romanini MV. Body image disorders and surgical timing in patients affected by poland syndrome: data analysis of 58 case studies. Plast Reconstr Surg. 2016;137(4):1273–82.
8. Romanini MV, Torre M, Santi P, Dova L, Valle M, Martinoli C, Baldelli I. Proposal of the TBN classification of thoracic anomalies and treatment algorithm for Poland syndrome. Plast Reconstr Surg. 2016;138(1):50–8.
9. Chavoin JP, Chaput B, Garrido I, Moreno B, Dahan M, Grolleau JL. [Correction of congenital malformations by custom-made silicone implants: Contribution of computer-aided design. Experience of 611 cases]. Ann Chir Plast Esthet. 2016;61(5):694–702.
10. Chavoin JP, Grolleau JL, Moreno B, Brunello J, André A, Dahan M, Garrido I, Chaput B. Correction of pectus excavatum by custom-made silicone implants: contribution of computer-aided design reconstruction. A 20-year experience and 401 cases. Plast Reconstr Surg. 2016;137(5):860e–71e.
11. Yiyit N, Işıtmangil T, Öksüz S. Clinical analysis of 113 patients with Poland syndrome. Ann Thorac Surg. 2015;99(3):999–1004.

12. Watfa W, di Summa PG, Raffoul W. Bipolar Latissimus Dorsi transfer through a single incision: First key-step in poland syndrome chest deformity. Plast Reconstr Surg Glob Open. 2016;4(8):e847.
13. Tvrdek M, Kletenský J, Svoboda S. Aplasia of the breast–reconstruction using a free tram flap. Acta Chir Plast. 2001;43(2):39–41.
14. Dos Santos Costa S, Blotta RM, Mariano MB, Meurer L, Edelweiss MI. Aesthetic improvements in Poland's syndrome treatment with omentum flap. Aesthetic Plast Surg. 2010;34(5):634–9.
15. Shamberger RC, Welch KJ, Upton J III. Surgical treatment of thoracic deformity in Poland's syndrome. J Pediatr Surg. 1989;24(8):760–5; discussion 766
16. Liao HT, Cheng MH, Ulusal BG, Wei FC. Deep inferior epigastric perforator flap for successful simultaneous breast and chest wall reconstruction in a Poland anomaly patient. Ann Plast Surg. 2005;55(4):422–6.
17. He J, Xu H, Wang T, Qiao Y, Zhang Y, Dong J. Immediate nipple reconstruction with thoracodorsal artery perforator flap in breast reconstruction by latissimus dorsi myocutaneous flap in patients with Poland's syndrome. Microsurgery. 2016;36(1):49–53.
18. Pinsolle V, Chichery A, Grolleau JL, Chavoin JP. Autologous fat injection in Poland's syndrome. J Plast Reconstr Aesthet Surg. 2008;61(7):784–91.
19. Chaput B, Mojallal A, Vaysse C, Lopez R, de Bonnecaze G. For the first time, a National Health Authority Provides Official Recommendations for autologous fat grafting in the breast. Plast Reconstr Surg. 2015;136(5):713e–4e.
20. Voglimacci M, Garrido I, Mojallal A, Vaysse C, Bertheuil N, Michot A, Chavoin JP, Grolleau JL, Chaput B. Autologous fat grafting for cosmetic breast augmentation: a systematic review. Aesthet Surg J. 2015;35(4):378–93.
21. Chaput B, Foucras L, Le Guellec S, Grolleau JL, Garrido I. Recurrence of an invasive ductal breast carcinoma 4 months after autologous fat grafting. Plast Reconstr Surg. 2013;131(1):123e–4e.
22. Perignon D, Marton A, Qassemyar Q, Carton S, Benhaim T, Morez B, Robbe M, Sinna R. [Custom made chest-wall implant and Poland's syndrome: between art and science]. Ann Chir Plast Esthet. 2010;55(3):225–32.
23. Del Frari B, Schwabegger AH. Clinical results and patient satisfaction after pectus excavatum repair using the MIRPE and MOVARPE technique in adults: 10-year experience. Plast Reconstr Surg. 2013;132:1591–602.

Breasts and Pectus Excavatum

5

Jean-Pierre Chavoin, Mary Morgan, Richard Vaucher,
Benjamin Moreno, Benoit Chaput,
and Jean-Louis Grolleau

5.1   Introduction

Pectus excavatum, or "funnel chest," is the most common congenital malformation of the thorax. In the literature, the sex ratio is mostly 5 men to 1 woman; in our 25-year experience of 600 cases, it was 3 men to 2 women owing to the quality of our plastic surgeon and the specific recruitment of breast anomalies due partly or totally to pectus excavatum.

In women, we can see specific deformations of the breasts (Fig. 5.1):

– With a varus or strabismus convergent in the medial and symmetrical forms
– With asymmetry, disorientation in varus, and a sagging breast located on the side of the lateral depression
– Breast hypotrophy can be associated, but it is safer to complete the treatment in a second procedure with classical silicone gel breast implants.

J.-P. Chavoin (✉) · B. Chaput · J.-L. Grolleau
Plastic Surgery Department, Rangueil Hospital, Toulouse University Hospital,
Toulouse, France
e-mail: jean-pierre.chavoin@orange.fr; chaput.b@chu-toulouse.fr; grolleau.jl@chu-toulouse.fr

M. Morgan
St Andrew's Centre for Plastic Surgery and Burns, Chelmsford, UK
e-mail: Mary.Morgan@meht.nhs.uk

R. Vaucher
Plastic and Reconstructive Surgery Department, Amiens Picardie University Hospital,
Amiens, France
e-mail: richard.vaucher@etud.u-picardie.fr

B. Moreno
AnatomikModeling, Amphipolis Business Centre, Toulouse, France
e-mail: bmoreno@anatomikmodeling.com

© Springer Nature Switzerland AG 2019
J.-P. Chavoin (ed.), *Pectus Excavatum and Poland Syndrome Surgery*,
https://doi.org/10.1007/978-3-030-05108-2_5

Fig. 5.1 Pectus affects the
breast shape in women
high convergence (type 1),
low convergence (type 2),
and asymmetry (type 3)

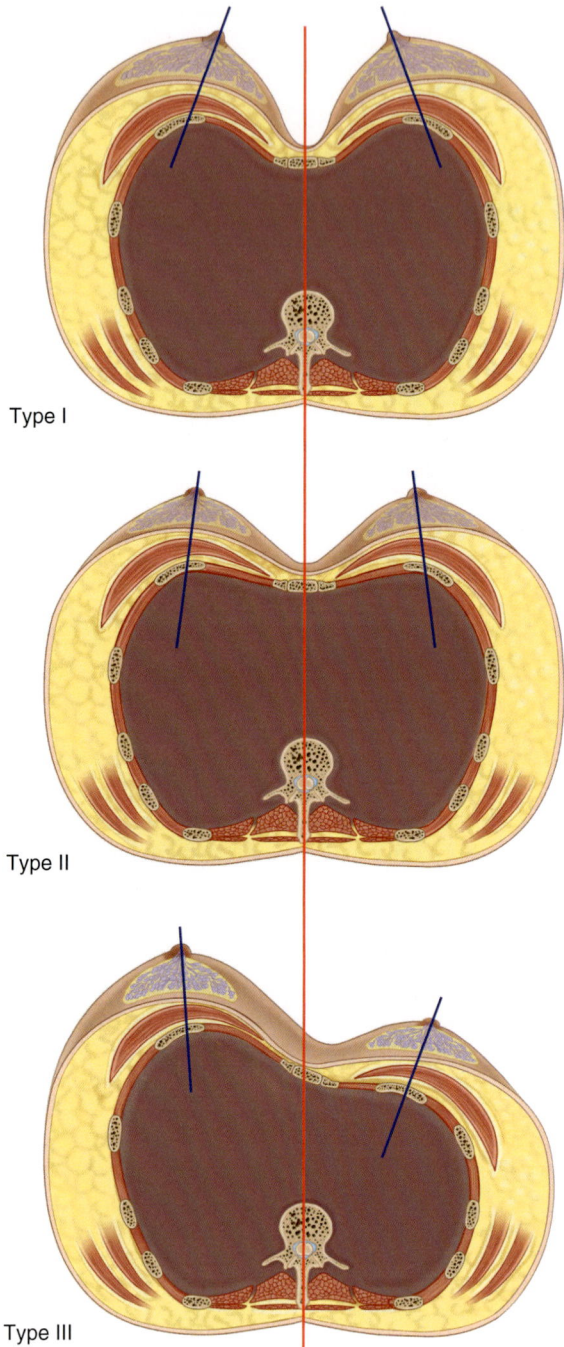

Type I

Type II

Type III

It is the breast deformity, asymmetry or hypotrophy that motivates the consultation, as the chest deformity is often unknown to the patient and her physician. For this reason, as plastic surgeons, we see more and more women with pectus and breast dystrophy.

5.2   Basic Principles

Thoracic deformity, even if it is severe, occasionally has functional repercussions (and again it is a decrease with no consequence of vital capacity). Respiratory functional exploration constantly shows this evidence, which should call into question any invasive orthopedic treatment aimed at reshaping the rib cage, whether Ravitch or Nuss sternochondroplasty in children and young patients (so-called minimally invasive technique). For this morphological disorder, the CAD silicone elastomer custom-made implant [1, 2] is the technique of choice (Fig. 5.2).

Chin's classification, which is simple and practical, distinguishes three types of pectus excavatum:

- Type 1 is deep, median, narrow, and symmetrical, with a large vertical axis
- Type 2 is wide, shallow, and symmetrical, with a large horizontal axis
- Type 3, significantly more common in women, is lateralized with rotation of the sternum

Fig. 5.2 Schematic illustration of pectus correction in a woman with a deep CAD custom-made elastomer silicone implant

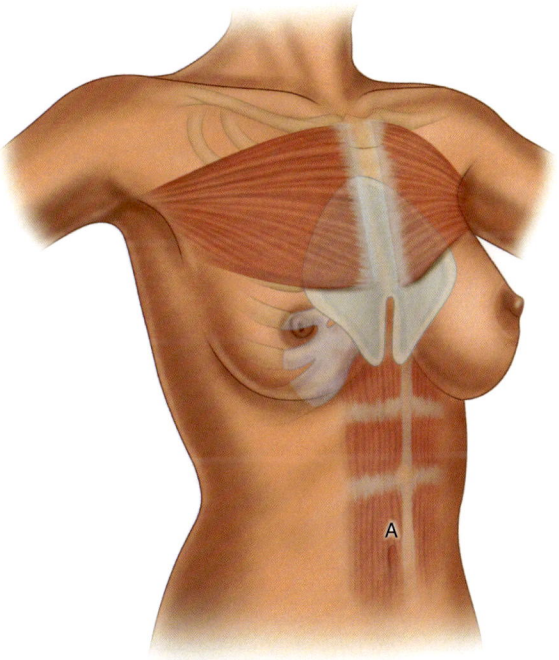

We added two other different types that we have encountered:

- Type 4 or pectus arcuatum, which associates a manubrial pectus carinatum and a pectus excavatum arched in the gladiolateral lower part of the sternum
- Type 5 secondary: poor results of other procedures such as Ravich, Nuss, pectus up, vacuum bell, and sometimes other traumas that occur in children during the course of growth.

All types cause a different breast deformity.

5.3   Custom-Made Implants in Women

Implantation of a precisely tailored molding of the anterior thorax through the use of Place of Zelgan® paste makes it possible to create a plaster mold, but the ideal (especially in women, with the presence of breasts) is a computer-aided design (CAD) from a 3D scanner. The first step is the computer reconstruction of the missing part of the thorax (Fig. 5.3); in the case of a woman, it largely overflows laterally behind the breasts to provide an antero-external projection that will correct the poor orientation in varus. In the case of asymmetry (type 3), it can compensate for

Fig. 5.3 3D computer image of an implant to correct asymmetrical breasts due to a Chin type 3 pectus excavatum

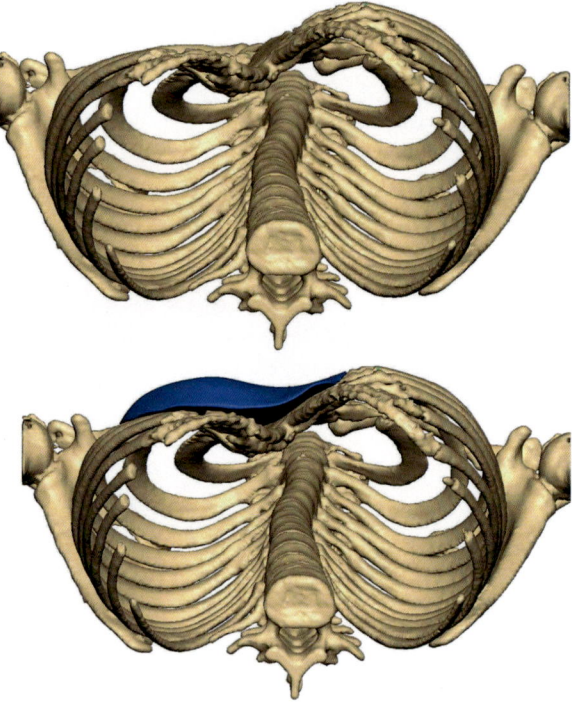

Fig. 5.4 CAD custom-made implant with a soft silicone elastomer just before being inserted to correct a type 3 pectus in a female patient

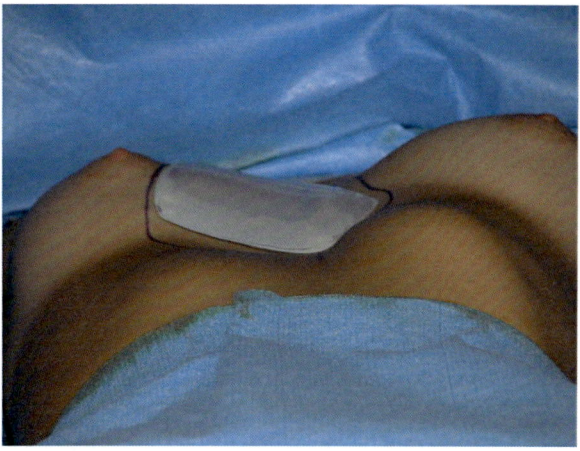

associated depression and hypotrophy. The image thus produced is transmitted to a prototyper, who makes a resin model using a 3D milling process. The prototype or model in resin is sent to the manufacturer, who must perform an implant in "gum" or silicone elastomer (Fig. 5.4). The implant must be both flexible, so that it can be introduced folded, solid, and does not tear. Chest deformity of any type can be corrected in this way.

5.4 Surgical Technique: Primary Pectus Correction

The procedure is performed under general anesthesia with intubation. The patient is placed supine, with the arms alongside the body.

5.4.1 Preoperative Drawing

This is the same as for men, but with breasts, the prototype is not perfectly adapted to the surface, as it is a CAD of the anterior thorax and not a plaster mold on the skin.

We draw the medial presternal line at an equal distance from the medial edge of both areolas, with the skin stretched. The incision is vertical, 6–8 cm long, centered at the deepest part of the deformation. We trace the exact contour of the prototype using a dermographic pencil, well positioned to mark the exact limits of the submuscular lodge and of the undermining. The good position of the implant is facilitated by the incrustation of a vertical line on the prototype (lateral control and rotation) and by a reference on the CAD to the exact distance between the sternal fork and the lower pole of the implant (height control). We must always refer to the computer image for the correct position of the implant and its lodge.

5.4.2   Incision

The skin incision is made with a scalpel and a section of the subcutaneous tissue sternal plan with an electric knife taking care not to burn the superficial skin edges by direct contact or through a metallic retractor.

5.4.3   Undermining

Lateral muscle detachment is bloodless; it ensures the progressive disinsertion of the medial attachments of the pectoralis major with electrocautery—easily at the level of its costal attachments, cautiously at the level of the intercostal spaces. Once past the muscle insertion zone, detachment is easier in the retromuscular cellular space and stops at the limits traced on the skin. The intervention is facilitated by the use an illuminated retractor or, better, a cold-light helmet. It is necessary to control the paramedian perforating vessels of the second and third intercostal spaces, which are sources of bleeding.

5.4.4   Caudal Detachment

Caudal detachment is performed using an electric knife, the anterior sheath of the rectus abdominis is transversely sectioned, 5 cm above the caudal limit, showing the underlying muscle. Subfascial and premuscular detachment is facilitated by the use of bipolar coagulation scissors, including the passage of the incisures; we retain the wall between the two rectus abdominis.

5.4.5   Implant Insertion

Through this narrow passage, we can put the implant in place folded in on itself. It then redeploys itself and takes its place spontaneously in the space and hollow. We control its good adaptation and position with the medial line. Drainage is not necessary. At its lower pole, the implant is cut vertically over 4 cm and inserted under the anterior sheath of the rectus abdominis, on both sides of the intermuscular septum. This stabilizes it, preventing possible displacement, particularly by avoiding a visible shift at the level of the epigastric area.

5.4.6   Closing

The closure is done in three planes with resorbable thread. The deep muscular plane is sutured in the cranial two thirds (Polysorb 0 large needle). The subcutaneous plane is sutured using reversed separated sutures (Monocryl® 3/0). The closure ends with a continuous intradermal suture (Monocryl® 3/0). External restraint is ensured by placement of a soft roll of Dacron® (Rolta) and a circular thoracic contention.

5.4.7   Postoperatively

The dressing and the restraint are maintained until the second day. A puncture of the sero-hematic effusion is quasi-systematic. A classical operative dressing is changed for a Mepilex border EM®. The patient can be administered analgesics and leave with a thoracic belt or a bra for effective compression. A large "hour glass"-shaped presternal pad maintains the breasts in a separate position, to respect the intermammary valley and avoid symmastia. A security control consultation is planned for the eighth day, without intermediate dressing. The punctures are made and renewed on request (two to three on average). Exercise cessation is recommended for 3 months to avoid muscular suture detachment.

5.4.8   Results and Complications

Whatever the type of malformation, the result must be a normal thorax and breasts; the implant must be invisible at the periphery owing to its fine edges and deep position. It is better to slightly hypocorrect rather than the opposite, which exposes the patient to an aspect in "plastron." Correction with a custom-made CAD elastomer implant improves the shape and dystrophy of the woman's chest, but the volume can also be made better because of the projection of the breast medially in type 1 (Fig. 5.5). In type 3, pure chest asymmetry, only a thoracic implant can provide perfect symmetry (Figs. 5.6 and 5.7). Type 3 with breast asymmetry is most frequent in women (50%).

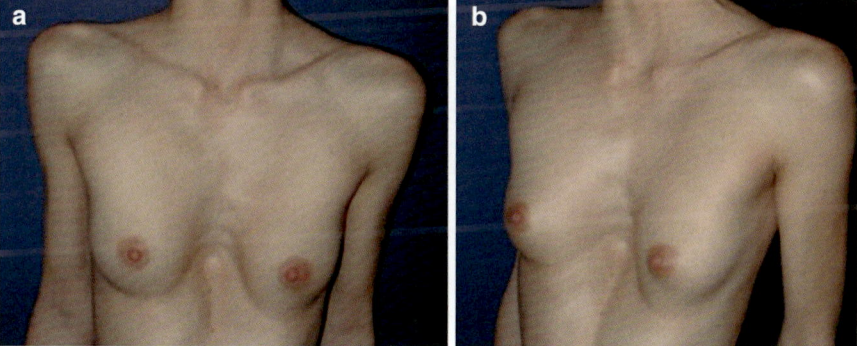

Fig. 5.5 Pectus excavatum, type 1, in a female patient. Result after 3 months. Note the dramatic result on the size of the breasts without breast implants. (**a**, **b**) Before, (**c**, **d**) 3 months after

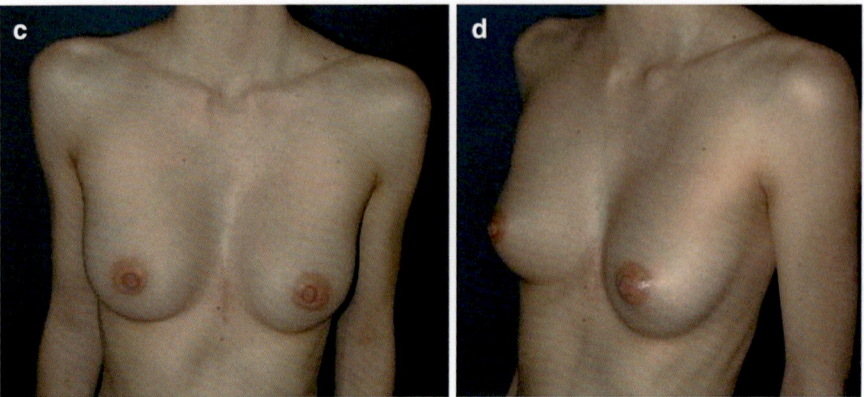

Fig. 5.5 (continued)

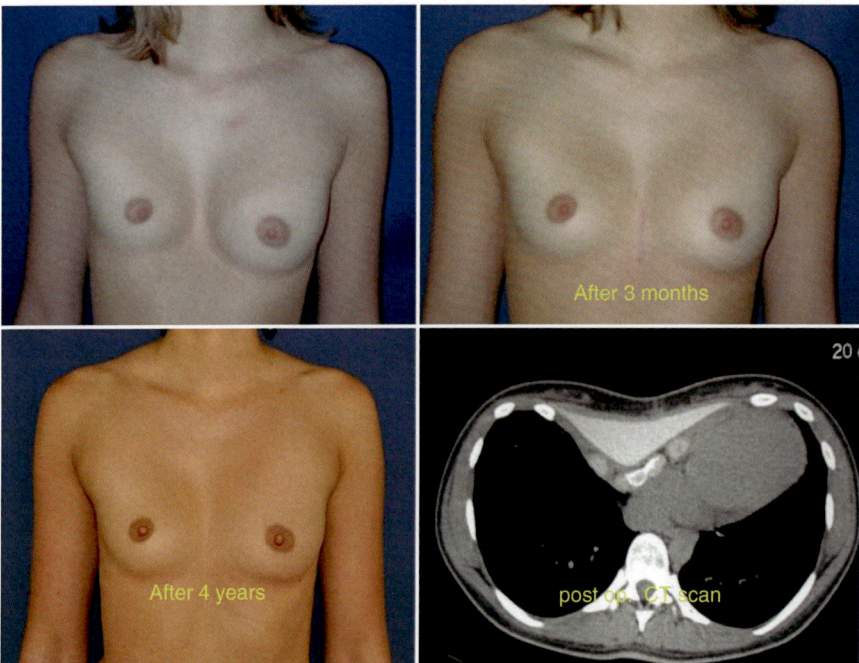

Fig. 5.6 Pectus excavatum type 3, deep, asymmetrical, in a female patient: the breast asymmetry is the result of the chest asymmetry. Thorax correction using a CAD custom-made implant results in perfect symmetry without any classic breast implant. Result after 3 months: scar is still reddish, but very discreet after 4 years

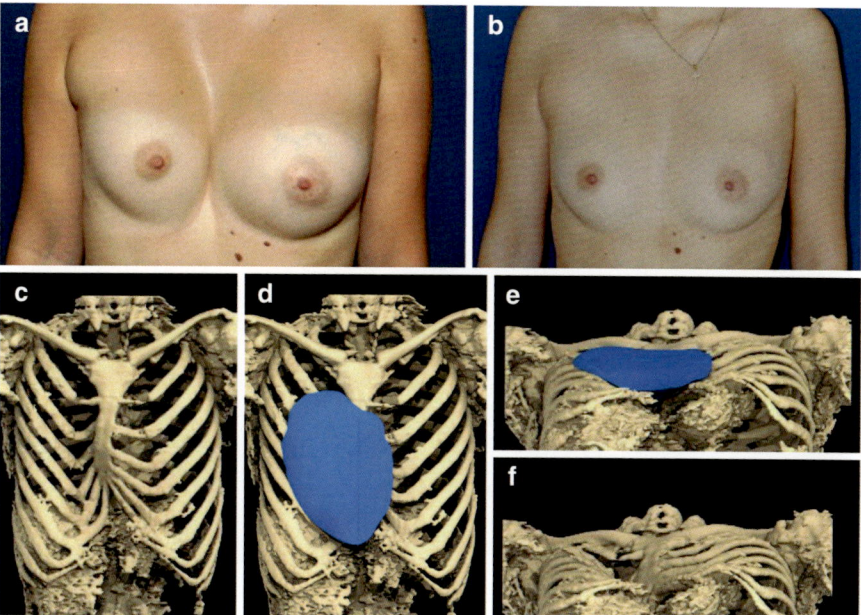

Fig. 5.7 Pectus excavatum type 3 with breast asymmetry in a female patient. (**a**) Before. (**b**) Result after 1 year. (**c**, **d**) Digital 3D image front facing and (**e**, **f**) supine view

The 6- to 8-cm presternal scar heals quickly, as closure is carried out without tension because of the excess cutaneous capital of the funnel, the medial muscle suture, and 1 month of compression.

The implant is retained for the rest of the patient's life, without management.

The fibrous encapsulation of the foreign body prevents any shifting or infection. There is neither contracture of the capsule nor rupture of the elastomer implant, as with classical silicone gel breast implants.

5.5 Surgical Technique: Secondary Breast Implants After Pectus Correction

In the case of hypotrophy of one breast associated with pectus, we first correct the pectus using a thoracic implant (Fig. 5.8). Implantation of one breast can be proposed, but only in a secondary procedure, after 6 months to 1 year and a good encapsulation of the first elastomer implant (Fig. 5.9). The same procedures as for bilateral breast hypotrophy are performed.

We always choose a submammary approach of 5 cm and a prepectoral position, so that the two implants can be separated by the muscle plane.

Breast & chest asymmetry

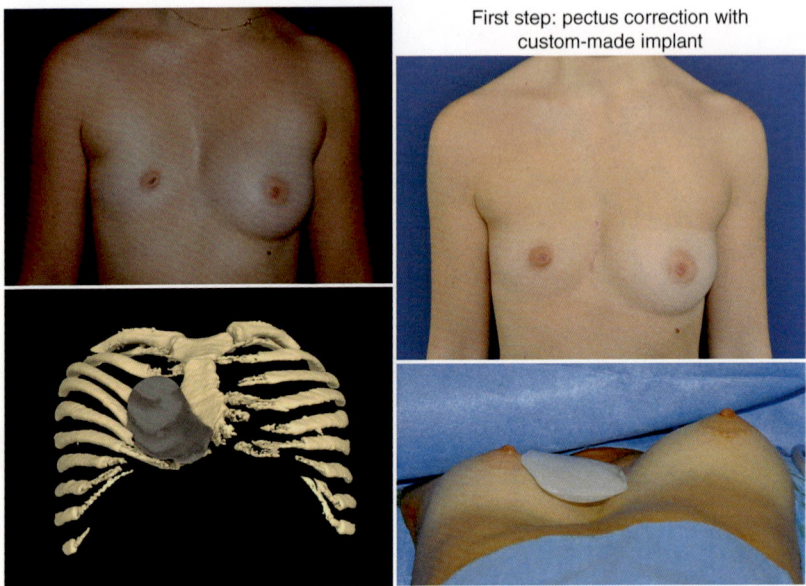

First step: pectus correction with custom-made implant

Fig. 5.8 Mixed thoracic and breast asymmetry. First step: pectus correction with custom-made implant

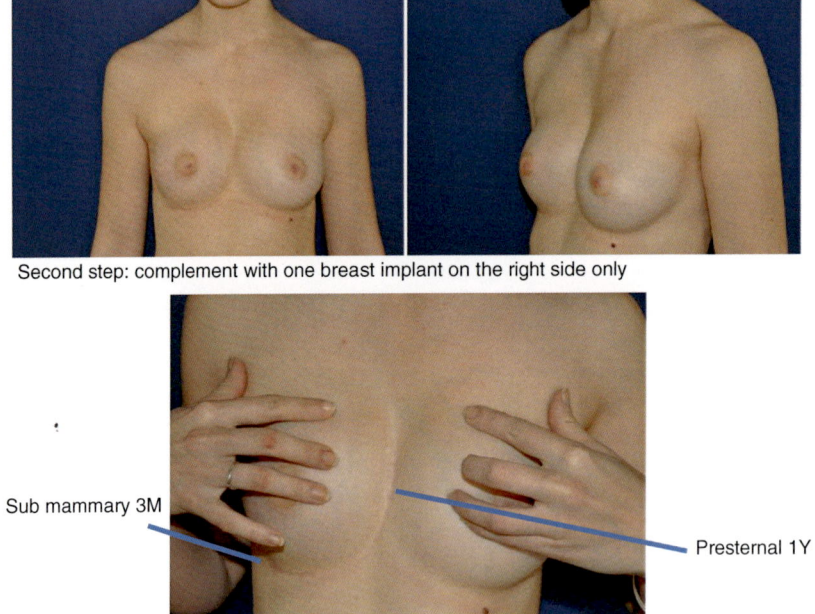

Second step: complement with one breast implant on the right side only

Sub mammary 3M

Presternal 1Y

Fig. 5.9 Second step: (1) complement with one breast implant on the right side after only 9 months. (2) Note the quality of the two scars: submammary on the right after 3 months, presternal after 1 year. Result after two breast implants inserted during a second procedure

5.6   Surgical Technique: Secondary Procedure After Primary Breast Implants

5.6.1   Temporary Ablation of the Breast Implants

Mostly, pectus excavatum correction with primary breast implants gives a poor result: either they accentuate the initial medial strabismus convergence of the breasts (Fig. 5.10) in type 1 or they cannot compensate for the asymmetry.

The best solution is to remove these breast implants, correct the pectus at the same time, and then insert new implants in a second procedure after 6 months or 1 year.

5.6.2   Retention of the Breast Implants and Thoracic Implant in the Same Procedure

In some rare cases, an elastomer implant can be inserted behind the breast implant if it has been placed in a pre-pectoralis position: it is easy to undermine behind the capsule; the position of the two breasts can be improved (Fig. 5.11).

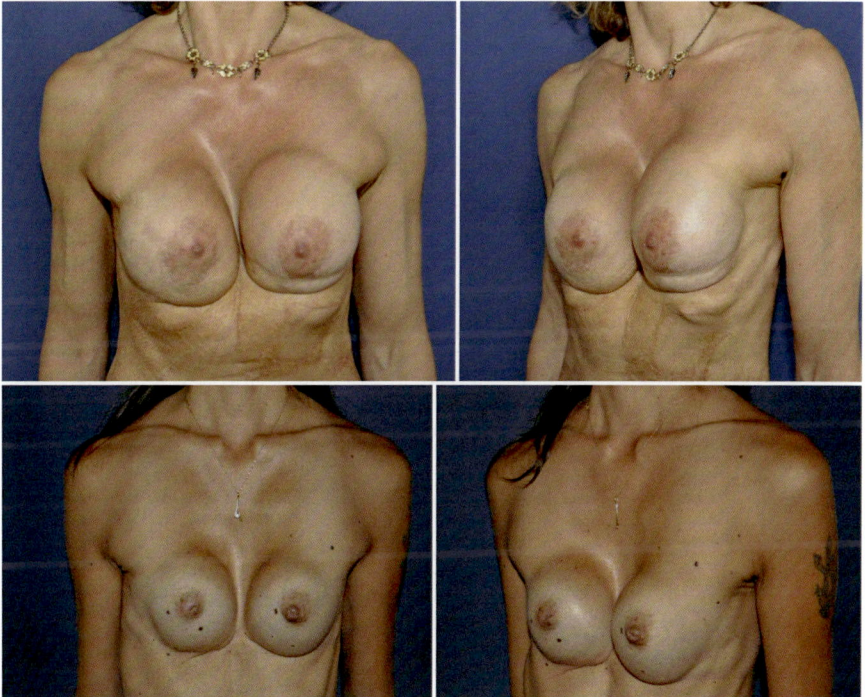

Fig. 5.10 Breast implants lead to increasing convergence if no previous correction of the pectus excavatum has been carried out

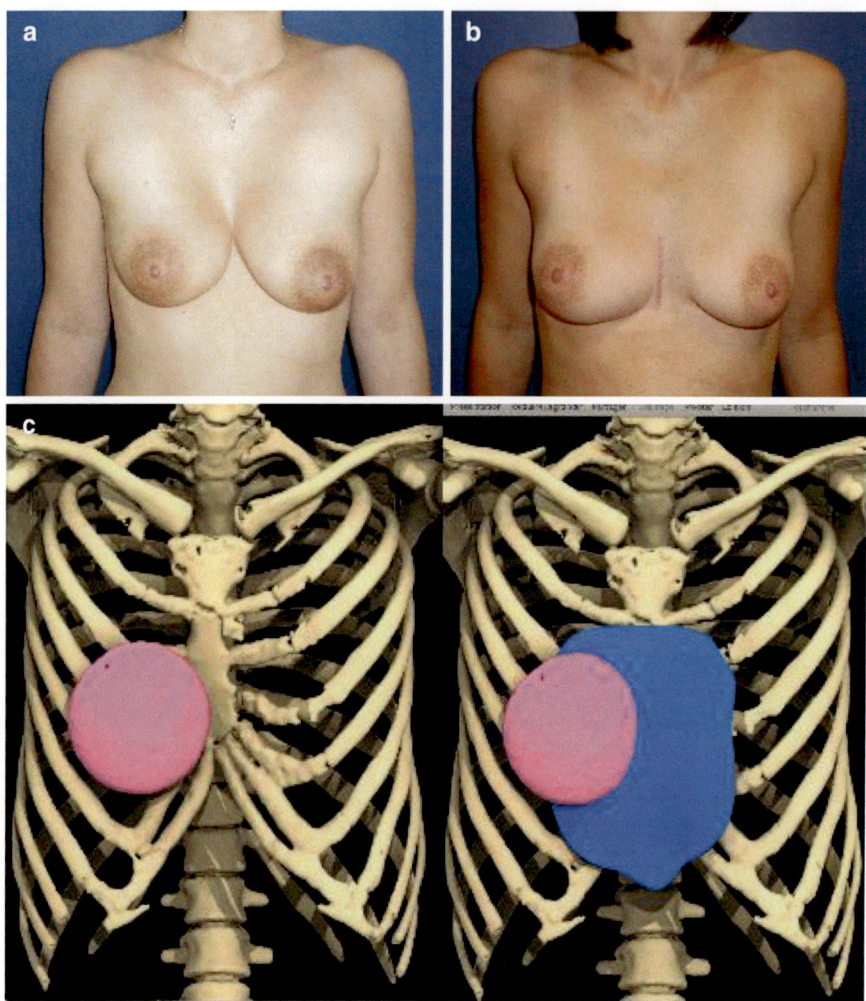

Fig. 5.11 (**a**) Breast asymmetry under-corrected with one right prepectoral implant. (**b**) Previous breast implant on the right can be maintained and a chest implant introduced behind the capsule. Note the good new orientation laterally. (**c**) 3D reconstruction: breast implant (pink), thoracic implant (blue)

If the previous breast implants have been inserted in a submuscular position, the deep undermining plane will open the capsule posteriorly and the elastomer thoracic implant will be laterally directly in contact with the other: there is a high risk of sliding and medial displacement of the gel breast implants. The medial part of the capsule must be preserved and strict medial binding with a large hourglass-shaped pad should be maintained for 2 months to retain the intermammary valley and avoid symmastia (Fig. 5.12).

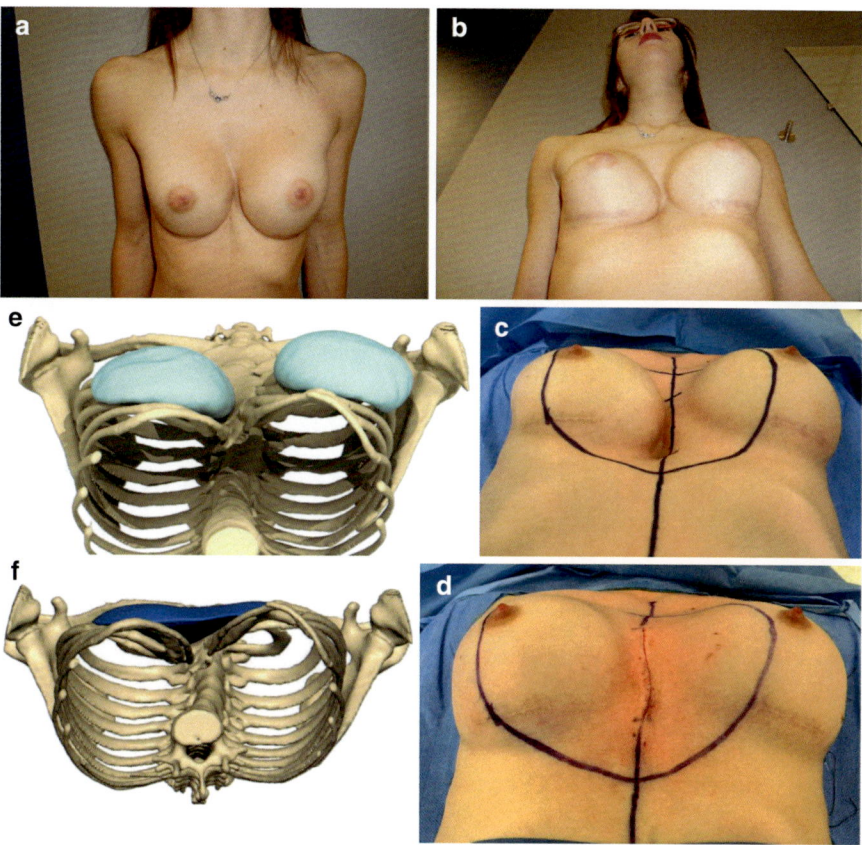

Fig. 5.12 CAD implant for the correction of pectus with previous breast implants inserted subpectorally (**a, b**) Preoperative view. (**c, d**) Per-operative view: implant is inserted behind the breast implants. (**e**) CAD with dystopic breast implants. (**f**) CAD thoracic implant

5.7   Surgical Technique: Secondary Procedure After Chin's Procedure

Chin's procedure is not a good choice, especially for young boys or girls with an asymmetric type 3 deformation: they always have a very painful postoperative period, a total restriction of sports activities for 3 years, and no proven functional benefit.

Pediatric surgeons are not in favor of the Nuss technique in the case of asymmetry.

5.7.1   Surgical Technique: Secondary Procedure After Chin's Bar Displacement

The bar must be removed by the pediatric or thoracic surgeon and then, after 6 months, a CAD custom-made silicone implant can be easily inserted using the same procedure: a presternal vertical approach and a submuscular position (Fig. 5.13).

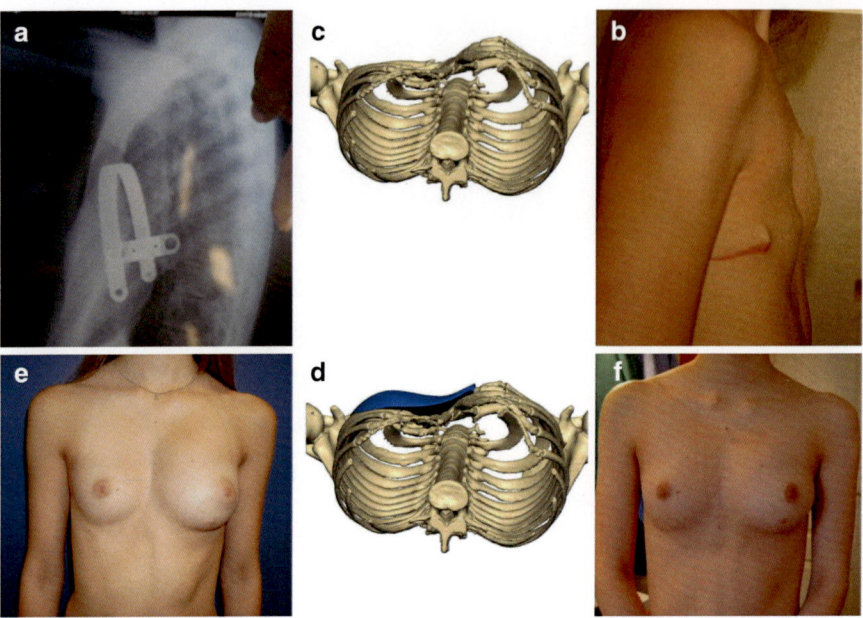

Fig. 5.13 (**a**, **b**) Failure of a Nuss procedure with bar rotation, (**c**, **d**) thoracic implant to correct asymmetry. (**e**) Before, (**f**) after

5.7.2   Surgical Technique: Secondary Procedure After a Poor Result with Chin's Procedure

After the Nuss procedure, removal of the bar (one to four in the case of bridges), the result may be inadequate or a partial recurrence may be observed in men and women.

It is easily and perfectly completed with a CAD custom-made silicone implant (Fig. 5.14).

5.8   Discussion

Many eminent plastic surgeons have published work on this nonfunctional congenital deformation and its direct implication for the shape and surgery of the breasts [3, 4].

The choice of a primary silicone gel breast implant to correct a pectus [5] is easier and cheaper, but exposes the patient to the risk of residual dystrophy owing to the worse orientation of the breasts after a volume augmentation on an incorrect thoracic base. This is true for any type of pectus, but especially in type 3, where a primary CAD custom-made implant has proved its effectiveness [6–8], after first attempts with molded plaster implants [9–11].

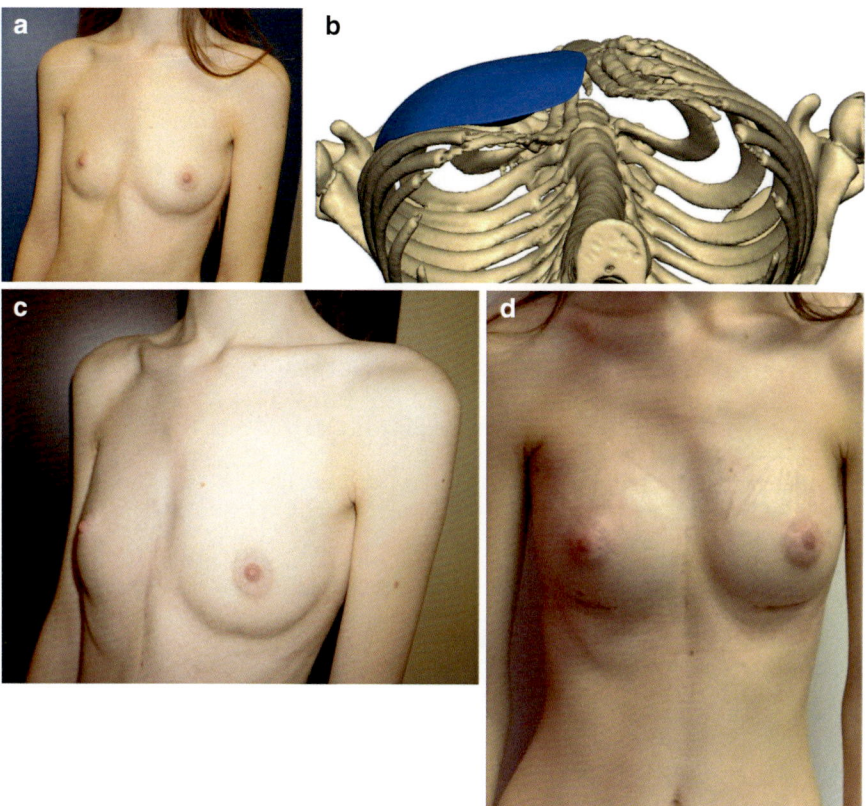

Fig. 5.14 (**a**) Failure of a Nuss procedure. Step 1: (**b, c**) thoracic implant to correct asymmetry. Step 2: (**d**) result after two breast implants inserted during a second procedure

The choice of an invasive procedure [12] is not suitable for this difficult anatomical context.

5.9 Conclusion

Breast deformities and asymmetries can be caused by an associated pectus excavatum.

Few physicians and surgeons have this knowledge and can provide a good orientation for an adapted treatment: a very precise morphological correction of the thorax by a silicone elastomer custom-made implant using CAD.

Plastic surgeons who try to correct these asymmetries with classic breast implants often have often poor results, sometimes worse than before.

In the case of breast hypotrophy associated with pectus excavatum, the first choice is to correct the shape of the thorax with a custom-made implant in a deep submuscular position; then, in a second procedure, place one or two breast implants via a submammary approach and in a premuscular position.

Invasive orthopedic procedures proposed by thoracic (Ravitch) and pediatric surgeons (Nuss) are not indicated in the absence of any functional problems, as they expose the patient to postoperative pain, sport restraint, complications, and at the very least a poor result, with often incomplete correction and deception.

There is no doubt for us that this type of treatment has a very low benefit–risk ratio and may now expose these specialists to medico-legal problems in the case of failure and lack of complete informed consent.

References

1. Chavoin JP. Plastic and reconstructive surgery of walls and borders [in French]. Paris: Elsevier Masson SAS Ed; 2009.
2. Chavoin JP. Plastic surgery of the breast [in French]. Paris: Elsevier Masson SAS Ed; 2011.
3. Bricout N. Chest morphology and breast augmentation [in French]. Ann Chir Plast Esthet. 2005;50:441–50.
4. Horch RE, Stoelben E, Carbon R, Sultan AA, Bach AD, Kneser U. Pectus excavatum breast and chest deformity: indications for aesthetic plastic surgery in a multicenter experience. Aesthet Plast Surg. 2006;30:403–11.
5. Moscona RA, Fodor L. How to perform breast augmentation safety for a pectus excavatum patient. Aesthet Plast Surg. 2011;35(2):198–202.
6. Ho Quoc C, Chaput B, Garrido I, Andre A, Grolleau J-L, Chavoin J-P. Management of breast asymmetry associated with primary funnel chest [in French]. Ann Chir Plast Esthet. 2013;58:54–9.
7. Chavoin J-P, Grolleau J-L, Moreno B, Brunello J, André A, Dahan M, et al. Correction of pectus excavatum by custom-made silicone implants: contribution of computer-aided design reconstruction. A 20-year experience and 401 cases. Plast Reconstr Surg. 2016;137(5):860e–71e.
8. Chavoin JP, André A, Bozonnet E, et al. Mammary implant selection or chest implants fabrication with computer help [in French]. Ann Chir Plast Esthet. 2010;55:471–80.
9. Hodgkinson DJ. The management of anterior chest wall deformity in patients presenting for breast augmentation. Plast Reconstr Surg. 2002;109:1714–23.
10. Hodgkinson DJ. Chest wall implants: their use for pectus excavatum, pectoralis muscle tears, Poland's syndrome, and muscular insufficiency. Aesthet Plast Surg. 1997;21:7–15.
11. Chavoin JP, Dahan M, Grolleau JL, Soubirac L, Wagner A, Foucras L, et al. Funnel chest: filling technique with deep custom made implant. Ann Chir Plast Esthet. 2003;48(2):67–76.
12. Fonkalsrud EW. Management of pectus chest deformities in female patients. Am J Surg. 2004;187:192–7.

Bibliography

1. Chavoin JP. Plastic and reconstructive surgery of walls and borders [in French]. Paris, France: Elsevier Masson SAS; 2009.
2. Hong JY, Suh SW, Park HJ, Kim YH, Park JH, Park SY. Correlations of adolescent idiopathic scoliosis and pectus excavatum. J Pediatr Orthop. 2011;31:870–4.
3. Malek MH, Berger DE, Marelich WD, Coburn JW, Beck TW, Housh TJ. Pulmonary function following surgical repair of pectus excavatum: a meta-analysis. Eur J Cardiothorac Surg. 2006;30:637–43.

 4. Guntheroth WG, Spiers PS. Cardiac function before and after surgery for pectus excavatum. Am J Cardiol. 2007;99:1762–4.
 5. Poupon M, Duteille F, Casanova D, Caye N, Magalon G, Pannier M. Pectus excavatum: what treatment in plastic surgery? About 10 cases [in French]. Ann Chir Plast Esthet. 2008;53:246–54.
 6. Bricout N. Chest morphology and breast augmentation [in French]. Ann Chir Plast Esthet. 2005;50:441–50.
 7. Chin EF, Adler RH. The surgical treatment of pectus excavatum. Br Med J. 1954;1:1064–6.
 8. Spear SL, Pelletiere CV, Lee ES, Grotting JC. Anterior thoracic hypoplasia: a separate entity from Poland syndrome. Plast Reconstr Surg. 2004;113:69–79.
 9. André A, Dahan M, Bozonnet E, Garrido I, Grolleau JL, Chavoin JP. Pectus excavatum: correction using the filling technique by a customized silicone implant in retromuscular position [in French]. In: Surgical techniques: plastic reconstructive and aesthetic surgery. Paris, France: EMC (Elsevier Masson SAS); 2010. p. 45–671. https://doi.org/10.1016/S1286-9325(10)46685-6.
10. Chavoin JP, André A, Bozonnet E, et al. Mammary implant selection or chest implants fabrication with computer help [in French]. Ann Chir Plast Esthet. 2010;55:471–80.
11. Médard de Chardon V, Balaguer T, Chignon-Sicard B, Ihrai T, Lebreton E. Constitutional asymmetries in aesthetic breast augmentation: incidence, postoperative satisfaction and surgical options [in French]. Ann Chir Plast Esthet. 2009;54:340–7.
12. Horch RE, Stoelben E, Carbon R, Sultan AA, Bach AD, Kneser U. Pectus excavatum breast and chest deformity: indications for aesthetic plastic surgery versus thoracic surgery in a multicenter experience. Aesthet Plast Surg. 2006;30:403–11.
13. Hodgkinson DJ. The management of anterior chest wall deformity in patients presenting for breast augmentation. Plast Reconstr Surg. 2002;109:1714–23.
14. Hodgkinson DJ. Chest wall implants: their use for pectus excavatum, pectoralis muscle tears, Poland's syndrome, and muscular insufficiency. Aesthet Plast Surg. 1997;21:7–15.
15. Beier JP, Weber PG, Reingruber B, et al. Aesthetic and functional correction of female, asymmetric funnel chest—a combined approach. Breast. 2009;18:60–5.
16. Fonkalsrud EW. Management of pectus chest deformities in female patients. Am J Surg. 2004;187:192–7.
17. Snel BJ, Spronk CA, Werker PM, van der Lei B. Pectus excavatum reconstruction with silicone implants longterm results and a review of the English-language literature. Ann Plast Surg. 2009;62:205–9.
18. Haecker FM. The vacuum bell for conservative treatment of pectus excavatum: the Basle experience. Pediatr Surg Int. 2011;27:623–7.
19. Pereira LH, Sterodimas A. Free fat transplantation for the aesthetic correction of mild pectus excavatum. Aesthet Plast Surg. 2008;32:393–6.
20. Delay E, Ho Quoc C, Garson S, Toussoun G, Sinna R. Autologous breast reconstruction by musculo-cutaneous-fatty pedicled latissimus dorsi flap [in French]. In: Surgical techniques: plastic reconstructive and aesthetic surgery. Paris, France: EMC (Elsevier Masson SAS); 2010. p. 45–665-C.
21. Delay E, Moutran M, Toussoun G, Ho Quoc C, Garson S, Sinna R. The role of fat transfer in breast reconstruction [in French]. In: Surgical techniques: plastic reconstructive and aesthetic surgery. Paris, France: EMC (Elsevier Masson SAS); 2011. p. 45–665-D.

Filling Method with Fat Graft Technique in Pectus Excavatum and Poland Syndrome

6

Christian Herlin

6.1 Introduction

Patients with pectus excavatum suffer from poor quality of life and impaired body image [1, 2]. The various existing surgical treatments have proven their efficacies in the treatment of this debilitating pathology in addition to improving the quality of life [3].

In addition to the techniques of chest wall bone remodeling, prosthetic filling techniques have largely shown their interest in the morphological correction of pectus excavatum and Poland syndrome. The contribution of CAD has been decisive in the progression of this technique, particularly for asymmetric and/or large pectus excavatum and especially in women, where the interfacing of the breasts causes preoperative conformation impairment [4–6].

Fat filling of breast asymmetries has been used for many years in malformative asymmetries or in post-tumorectomy/mastectomy sequelae [7, 8]. Also, it is currently one of the main tools used for the symmetrization of the breast of young women with Poland syndrome [9, 10]. The use of adipocyte autograft for the filling of pectus excavatum is more recent and does appear to be reserved for pectus excavatum of very low severity [11, 12]. Hyaluronic acid injection has also been proposed as an alternative to fat with interesting results [13].

We started using lipofilling as a supplement or alternative or other techniques for 6 years. After recalling the operating principles, we will detail our results on a consecutive single-center series of 28 patients.

C. Herlin (✉)
Plastic and Reconstructive Surgery Department, Lapeyronie Hospital,
Montpellier University Hospital, Montpellier, France
e-mail: c-herlin@chu-montpellier.fr

© Springer Nature Switzerland AG 2019
J.-P. Chavoin (ed.), *Pectus Excavatum and Poland Syndrome Surgery*,
https://doi.org/10.1007/978-3-030-05108-2_6

6.2   Operative Technique

6.2.1   Fat Harvesting

Fat is generally harvested under anesthesia. Most of the patients in our series had a small amount of fat, which led us to take up fat in all storage areas (thighs, loins, abdomen, etc.). Before harvesting, donor sites are infiltrated with serum mixed with epinephrine. Usually, we have infiltrated the same amount of serum that we had planned to take from fat to increase the volume of the fatty tissue through hydro-dissection and thus to reduce the intervention time and blood loss. At the end of the procedure, donor sites are infiltrated with local anesthetic. Fat harvesting is carried out with a specific cannula (diameter: 3 mm (8G), length: 15 cm) fixed on 10 mL LuerLock® type syringe. Harvested fat is then purified according to the method described by Sinna et al. [7].

The fat-filled syringes are centrifuged at 3000 rpm/min during 3 min to obtain three distinct layers:

– The oily upper layer consists of products of adipocyte degradation.
– The reddish bottom layer corresponds to products of hematic degradation.
– The middle layer corresponds to the fat to be injected.

On average, for each 100 mL of harvested fat tissue, about 30 mL is waste that is not used for injection (Fig. 6.1).

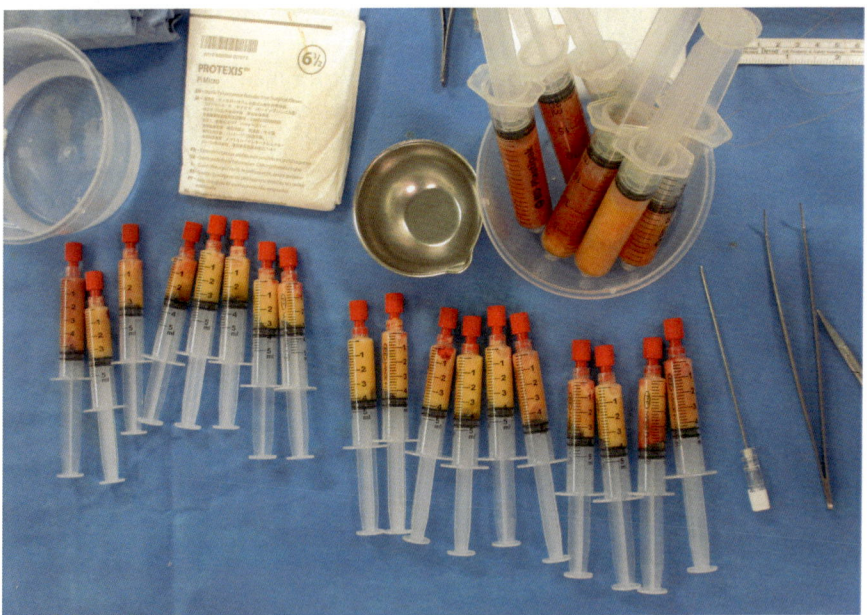

Fig. 6.1 Fat-filled syringes after centrifugation: middle layer (70%) corresponds to the fat to be injected. Oil and blood are wasted

6.2.2   Fat Grafting

Fat is injected using a specific 18G cannula through a stab incision made with an 18G trocar. Fat is grafted from the bottom of the target site towards the surface while withdrawing the cannula (Fig. 6.2). Fat placement follows the concentric circles that mark the deformity contour and that were drawn with the patient in standing position and under incident light before the intervention (Fig. 6.3). Fat should be placed in order to form a three-dimensional scaffold to increase the

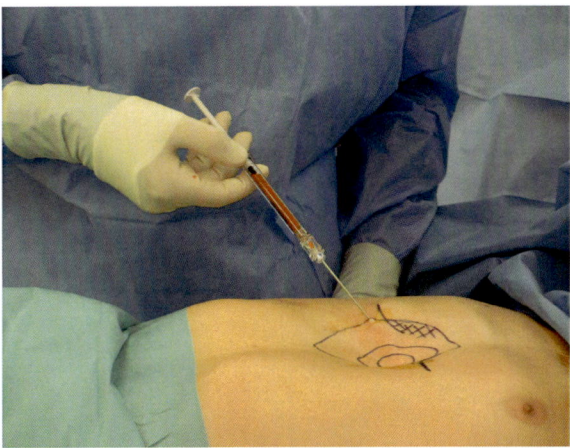

Fig. 6.2 Cannula is withdrawn from the bottom of the target site, towards the surface

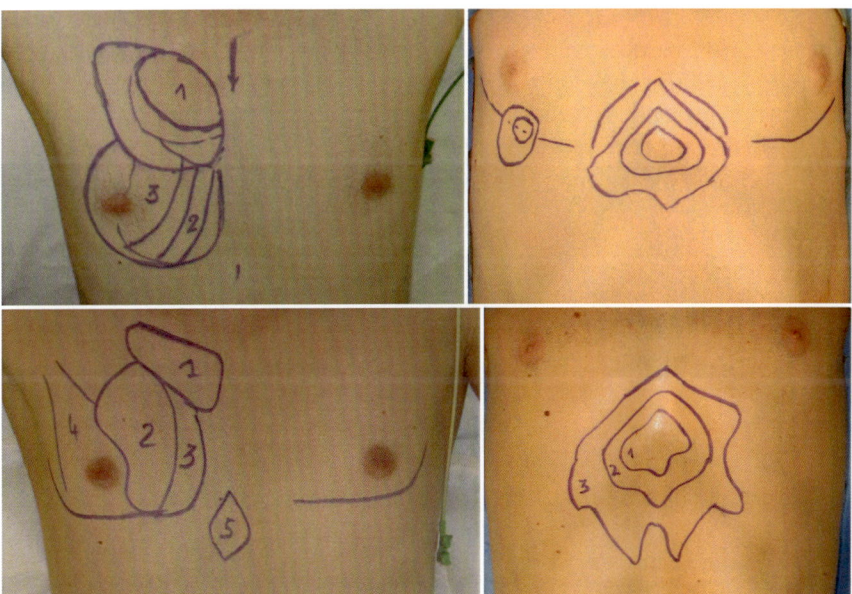

Fig. 6.3 Fat placement follows the concentric circles that mark the deformity contour (Poland left, Pectus right)

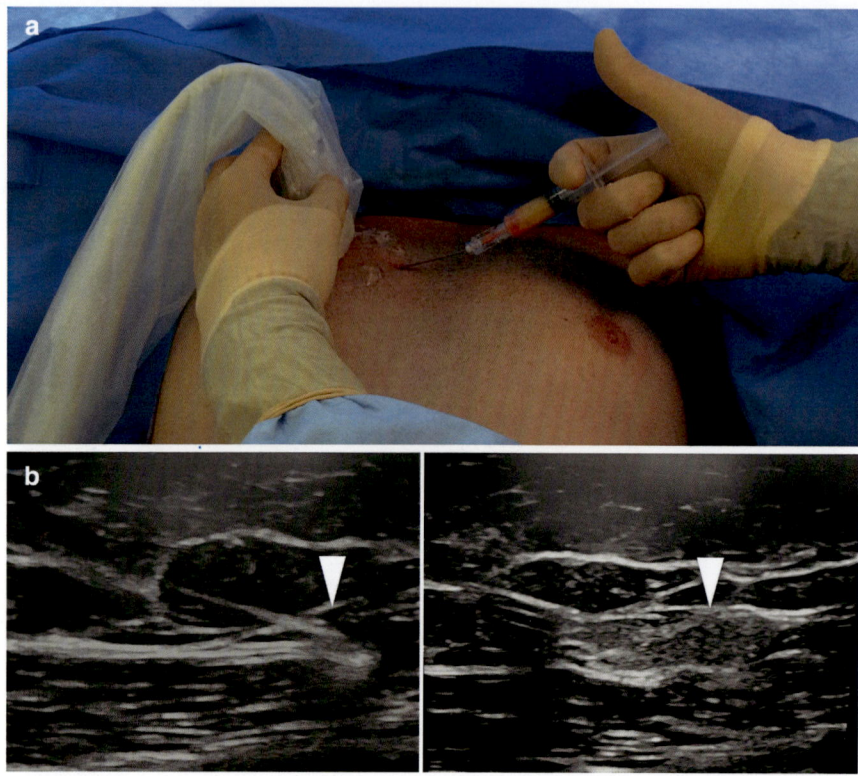

Fig. 6.4 (**a**) Intraoperative ultrasound. (**b**) echo control of the intramuscular injections

contact surface between adipocytes and the recipient tissue. The use of intraoperative ultrasound (Fig. 6.4a) allows intramuscular injection (Fig. 6.4b) in some very asymmetric shapes, which enables the surgeon to redraw the contours and maintain the fat graft in a more localized area.

Post-operative care is very simple. Ice packs can be applied to the donor site, but not the recipient site. Low-grade pain-killers are usually enough. Patients can walk the day after surgery and the procedure is generally carried out as ambulatory surgery.

6.3   Case Series

6.3.1   Pectus Excavatum (Table 6.1)

In the last 6 years, we have used lipofilling in the treatment of pectus excavatum in 28 patients. The average age of patients was 32 years old. They were mainly men (*n* = 23). The pectus was deep centered and narrow (Chin type 1, Fig. 6.5) in 6 patients, whereas it was wide centered and shallow (Chin type 2, Fig. 6.6) in 11

Table 6.1 Clinical data of our cohort

	Age	Genre	Chin type	Primary/secondary procedure	Nb of procedures	Total volume injected	Complications	Self-evaluation score	Late silicone implant correction
1	48	F	1	Secondary (Breast implants)	1	60	None	Failed	Yes
2	22	M	2	Primary	2	220	None	Good	No
3	38	M	3	Primary	2	180	None	Excellent	No
4	25	M	2	Primary	1	100	None	Good	No
5	45	M	3	Primary	1	180	None	Good	No
6	35	M	1	Primary	3	340	None	Excellent	No
7	42	M	2	Primary	1	80	None	Failed	Yes
8	22	F	3	Secondary (Sternochondroplasty)	1	90	None	Good	N/A
9	30	M	1	Primary	1	80	None	Good	No
10	19	M	2	Primary	2	160	None	Failed	No
11	28	F	3	Secondary (Sternochondroplasty)	1	100	None	Good	N/A
12	42	M	3	Primary	2	130	None	Good	No
13	48	M	1	Primary	2	260	None	Excellent	No
14	26	M	3	Secondary (Nuss)	3	370	None	Excellent	No
15	39	M	2	Primary	2	210	None	Good	Yes
16	24	M	2	Primary	1	180	None	Good	No
17	34	M	2	Primary	2	200	None	Failed	No
18	25	M	2	Secondary (Nuss)	1	170	None	Excellent	N/A
19	17	M	1	Primary	1	120	None	Good	No
20	32	M	3	Primary	2	190	None	Excellent	No
21	20	M	3	Secondary (Nuss)	3	350	None	Excellent	N/A
22	34	M	3	Primary	2	220	None	Excellent	No
23	21	M	2	Primary	2	200	None	Good	No
24	42	M	1	Primary	1	130	None	Good	No
26	37	M	3	Primary	2	210	None	Good	No
27	33	F	2	Secondary (Sternochondroplasty)	1	200	None	Excellent	N/A
28	41	M	2	Primary	2	190	None	Good	No

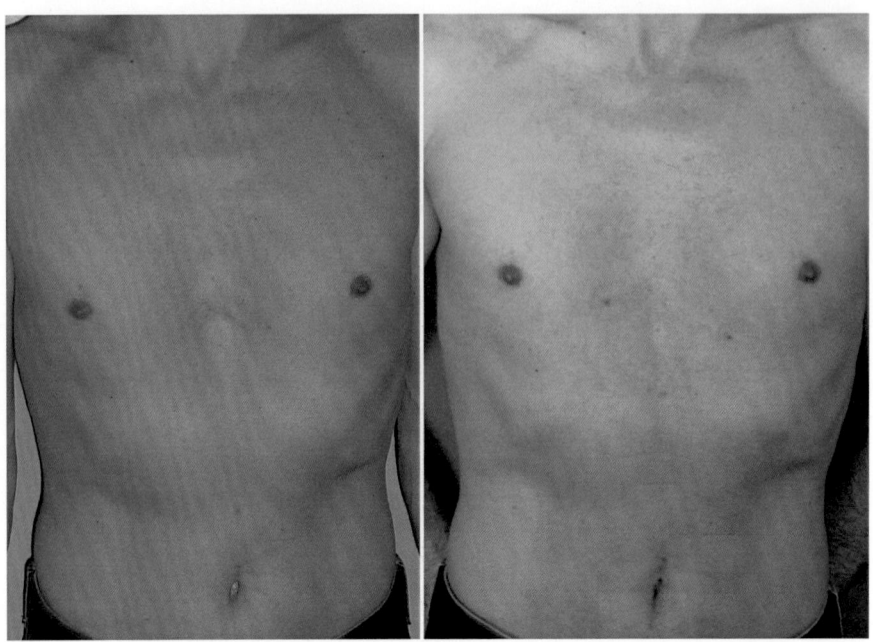

Fig. 6.5 Chin type 1 pectus before and after lipofilling

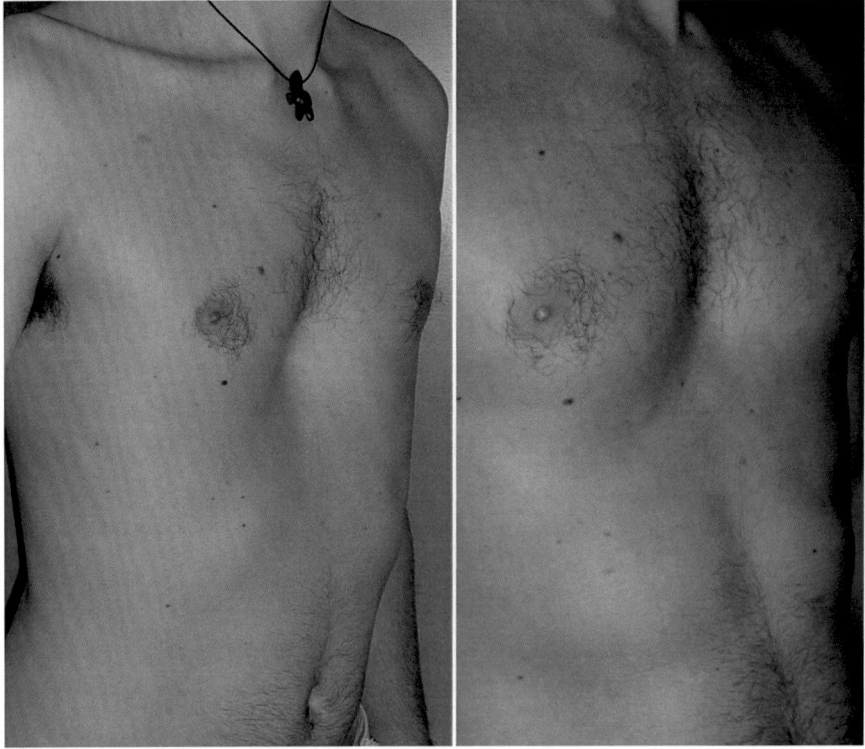

Fig. 6.6 Chin type 2 pectus before and after lipofilling

patients and finally lateralized (Chin type 3) in 11 other patients. The filling was followed by sternochondroplasty or Nuss surgery in seven cases (25%), whereas it was primitive in 75% of cases. The average number of procedures per patient was 1.7 and the average volume injected per patient was 182 cm³.

No complications at the donor or grafted site were noted in the 28 operated patients.

Patients surveyed at 3 months post-op rated the correction Excellent in 32% of cases (9/28), Good in 50% (14/28), and finally found the result Failed in 14% of cases (4/28). An obvious resorption was observed in 11 patients (39%) without it being objectively quantified. This resorption led to an additional procedure in four cases (13%). Thirteen percent of treated patients (4/23) had recourse to silicone elastomer implant correction due to insufficient result.

6.3.2 Poland Syndrome

We have used lipofilling as a solution for thoracic and breast symmetrization of Poland syndrome in five cases over the last 6 years. All of our interested treated cases of young women (average age 24.4 years, 17–34).

In three cases, it was the additional projection of segments 1 and 2 after placement of the breast prostheses when we had not used a thoracic silicone elastomer prosthesis. The principle was always to fill the depressed subclavicular region and the junction of segments 1 and 2 which is still in our very angular experience after placement of prosthesis (Fig. 6.7).

In two cases, we intended to symmetrize the breasts after placement of silicone elastomer prosthesis when the residual hypoprojection of the breast was small.

Regarding the first indications, we were most often led to perform two procedures (average: 1.67 interventions per patient). Regarding the second indication, we had realized only one injection to get the satisfaction of the patients.

6.4   Conclusions

Adipocyte autograft is a safe and controlled technique for the majority of reconstructive surgery teams that support pectus excavatum and Poland syndrome. We believe that this technique should be an integral part of the therapeutic arsenal of primary treatment of pectus excavatum of mild severity and in retouching sternochondroplasties, Nuss techniques, or prosthesis placement when the peripheral outcome is incomplete. Regarding the treatment of Poland syndrome, lipofilling is an essential tool in the correction of breast and thoracic asymmetry in addition to custom-made silicone implant. This option has multiple advantages: autologous material, ambulatory surgery, absence of scarring, and little risk of infection.

The resorption remains difficult to predict and the presence of a low BMI population in this pathology represents the main limitations of this safe and reproducible technique.

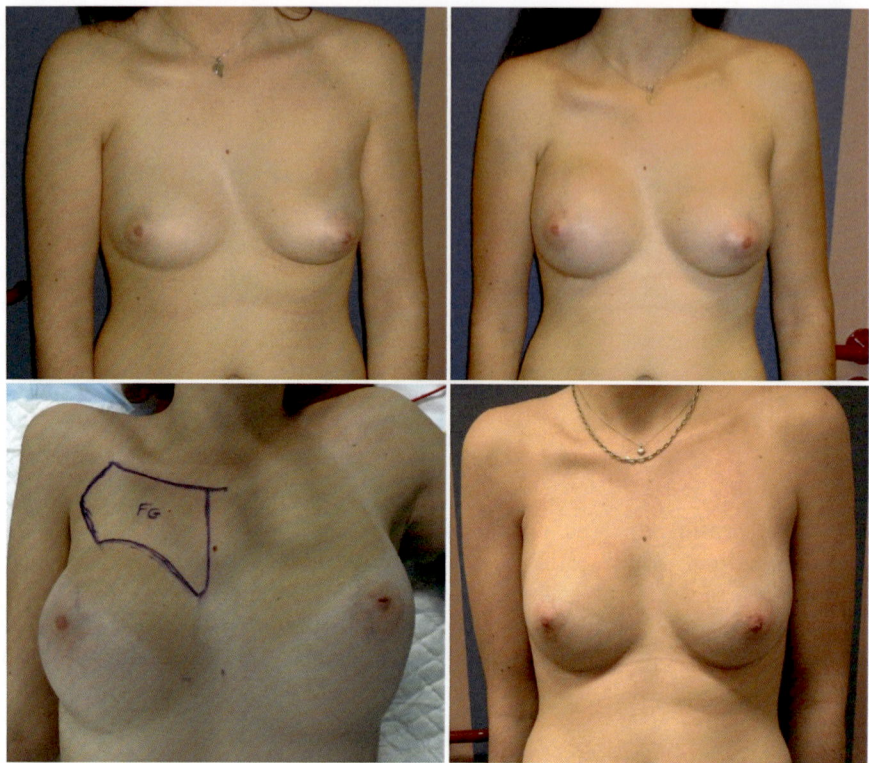

Fig. 6.7 Right Poland syndrome on a female: subclavicular filling after breast implant

References

1. Krille S, Muller A, Steinmann C, Reingruber B, Weber P, Martin A. Self- and social perception of physical appearance in chest wall deformity. Body Image. 2012;9:246–52.
2. Steinmann C, Krille S, Mueller A, Weber P, Reingruber B, Martin A. Pectus excavatum and pectus carinatum patients suffer from lower quality of life and impaired body image: a control group comparison of psychological characteristics prior to surgical correction. Eur J Cardiothorac Surg. 2011;40:1138–45.
3. Kelly RE Jr, Cash TF, Shamberger RC, Mitchell KK, Mellins RB, Lawson ML, Oldham K, Azizkhan RG, Hebra AV, Nuss D, Goretsky MJ, Sharp RJ, Holcomb GW III, Shim WK, Megison SM, Moss RL, Fecteau AH, Colombani PM, Bagley T, Quinn A, Moskowitz AB. Surgical repair of pectus excavatum markedly improves body image and perceived ability for physical activity: multicenter study. Pediatrics. 2008;122(6):1218–22.
4. Chavoin JP, André A, Bozonnet E, Teisseyre A, Arrue J, Moreno B, et al. Apport de l'informatique à la sélection des implants mammaires ou à la fabrication sur mesure des implants thoraciques. Annales De Chirurgie Plastique Esthétique. 2010;55(5):471–80. https://doi.org/10.1016/j.anplas.2010.08.002.
5. Chavoin J-P, Grolleau JL, Moreno B, Brunello J, André A, Dahan M, et al. Correction of pectus excavatum by custom-made silicone implants. Plast Reconstr Surg. 2016;137(5):860e–71e.

6. Ellart J, François C, Calibre C, Guerreschi P, Duquennoy-Martinot V. Asymétrie mammaire de l'adolescente et de la jeune adulte. Stabilité du résultat dans le temps. À propos de 144 patientes. Annales De Chirurgie Plastique Esthétique. 2016;61(5):665–79.
7. Sinna R, Delay E, Garson S, Delaporte T, Toussoun G. Breast fat grafting (lipomodelling) after extended latissimus dorsi flap breast reconstruction: a preliminary report of 200 consecutive cases. Br J Plast Surg. 2010;63(11):1769–77. https://doi.org/10.1016/j.bjps.2009.12.002.
8. Agha RA, Fowler AJ, Herlin C, Goodacre TE, Orgill DP. Use of autologous fat grafting for breast reconstruction: a systematic review with meta-analysis of oncological outcomes. J Plast Reconstr Aesthet Surg. 2015;68(2):143–61. https://doi.org/10.1016/j.bjps.2014.10.038.
9. Pinsolle V, Chichery A, Grolleau JL, Chavoin JP. Autologous fat injection in Poland's syndrome. J Plast Reconstr Aesthet Surg. 2008;61(7):784–91. https://doi.org/10.1016/j.bjps.2007.11.033.
10. Delay E, La Marca S, Guerid S. Correction de la déformation thoracomammaire du syndrome de Poland. Annales De Chirurgie Plastique Esthétique. 2016;61(5):652–64. https://doi.org/10.1016/j.anplas.2016.07.011.
11. Pereira LH, Sterodimas A. Free fat transplantation for the aesthetic correction of mild pectus excavatum. Aesthet Plast Surg. 2008;32(2):393–6. https://doi.org/10.1007/s00266-007-9110-x.
12. Ho Quoc C, Delaporte T, Meruta A, La Marca S, Toussoun G, Delay E. Breast asymmetry and pectus excavatum improvement with fat grafting. Aesthet Surg J. 2013;33(6):822–9. https://doi.org/10.1177/1090820X13493907.
13. Sinna R, Pérignon D, Assaf N, Berna P. Use of macrolane to treat pectus excavatum. Ann Thorac Surg. 2012;93(1):e17–8. https://doi.org/10.1016/j.athoracsur.2011.09.054.

Ian Hunt and Stephanie Fraser

7.1 Introduction

Pectus excavatum is the most common congenital chest wall deformity affecting 1 in 300–400 births. Patients typically describe a combination of physical and psychological symptoms relating to their deformity which can be debilitating for this young patient population. Surgical correction of the underlying chest wall deformity through internal bracing (MIRPE, minimally invasive repair of pectus excavatum or the Nuss procedure) or through a 'break and re-set' of the chest wall (modified Ravitch procedure) remains an important option in treating pectus excavatum particularly in the context of functional impairment.

7.2 Clinical Findings

Patients present with abnormal elongation and deformity of the hyaline costal cartilage of the anterior ribcage, resulting in depression of the sternum. This may or may not be associated with asymmetry and sternal angulation or rotation.

Though often described as congenital and therefore present at birth, it is more typical for patients with pectus excavatum to notice the sternal depression in the pre-teen years and particularly early teens as it worsens with growth. A family history is often noted.

Symptoms associated with pectus excavatum typically include breathlessness, chest pain or discomfort, pre-syncope or syncope particularly on exertion and

I. Hunt (✉)
Pectus Clinic, London, UK
e-mail: enquires@pectusclinic.com

S. Fraser
Guy's Hospital, London, UK
e-mail: stephanie.fraser3@nhs.net

© Springer Nature Switzerland AG 2019
J.-P. Chavoin (ed.), *Pectus Excavatum and Poland Syndrome Surgery*,
https://doi.org/10.1007/978-3-030-05108-2_7

Table 7.1 Symptoms associated with pectus excavatum

Symptom	Characteristic
Pain	Noted in the chest and back area, tends to come and go and may be made worse by certain activities and exercises. May be worse during periods of excessive growth. Poor posture may aggravate
Breathlessness	Sensation of shortness of breath, tight chestiness, constriction of breathing, often worse on certain activities and exercises
Palpitations	In severe forms, with heart distortion, there may be an increased incidence of heart palpitations
Fainting	Rarely, in severe pectus excavatum, feeling faint (pre-syncope) or actually fainting (syncope) can occur classically during exercise and is thought to be caused by distortion of the heart from the indrawn sternum
Psychological	Can have significant impact on a patient's self-esteem and confidence

palpitations (Table 7.1). Patients may also describe limitations to their exercise tolerance and fatigue when compared with their peers [1].

Often termed 'pectus posture', this refers to a combination of musculoskeletal abnormalities apparent in some patients with pectus deformity. It includes forward protruding head and neck, rounded and occasionally uneven shoulders (protruding anteriorly), thoracic kyphosis as well as an association with thoracic scoliosis and anterior pelvic tilt with a 'pot' belly. Often described as an 'attempt' to hide the pectus deformity, it is the senior author's belief that it is more a physiological response to the pectus deformity.

From a psychological perspective, there are high rates of social anxiety and depression in this patient group. Much of the decision-making around treatment should be focused on assessing the patient's psychological concerns. Surgical correction has been shown in patients with mental health concerns prior to surgery to alleviate those concerns [2].

7.3   Patient Selection

The decision to offer surgical correction is largely based on the severity of the deformity, patient choice including the psychosocial impact and physical impairment of the deformity. In patients with symptoms, further investigations should be considered to identify patients with pectus excavatum associated with functional impairment. In addition, relative contraindications to surgical correction include complex congenital anomalies including primary cardiac and pulmonary impairment and neurodevelopmental disorders.

7.3.1   Severity

Whilst many patients may be offered surgery on the basis of a clinical assessment of severity of the deformity, the severity can also be quantified by calculating the Haller index (HI). This is a comparison of the width of the thoracic cavity to the depth between the sternum and the spine on computer tomography (CT). Alternatives to a CT now include a rapid MRI (magnetic resonance imaging) protocol and 3D topographic body scanning which minimise the radiation exposure in this young patient population. Typically, a Haller index of >3.25 is considered an indication for surgery; however, this may be augmented by a correction index (CI) which accounts for abnormal chest morphologies [3]. The correction index unlike the Haller index which relies on the width of the chest wall appears more accurate in non-standard chest morphologies. A CI >28% correlates with a Haller index of >3.25 (Fig. 7.1).

7.3.2 Patient Choice

Patients will often be driven to seek correction of their deformity based on the severity of their symptoms (both physical and psychological) rather than the severity of the deformity itself. In young patients, it is important to elucidate their wishes as opposed to those of their parents. It is also essential to consider whether patients

Fig. 7.1 Image of CT scan of a pectus patient showing: (**a**) Haller index, a measurement of the internal transverse diameter of the thorax on the inside of the ribcage (in red), divided by the shortest anteroposterior depth from the internal aspect of the sternum of the anterior cortex of the nearest vertebral body (in blue). (**b**) Corrective index is the ratio of the anticipated rise in the sternal defect (in red) after bar placement (*a*), to the shortest anteroposterior dimension of the inner chest (*b*), multiplied by 100. It does not rely on the transverse diameter of the chest

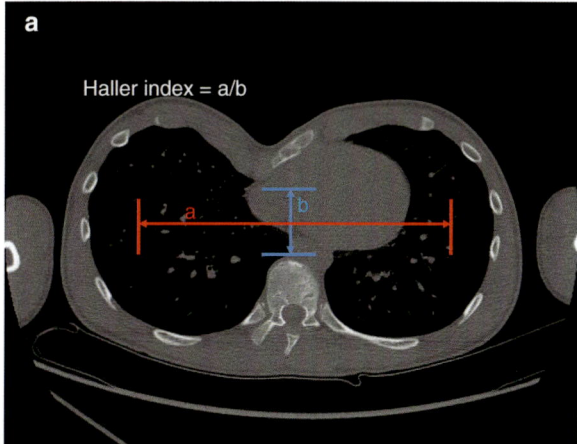

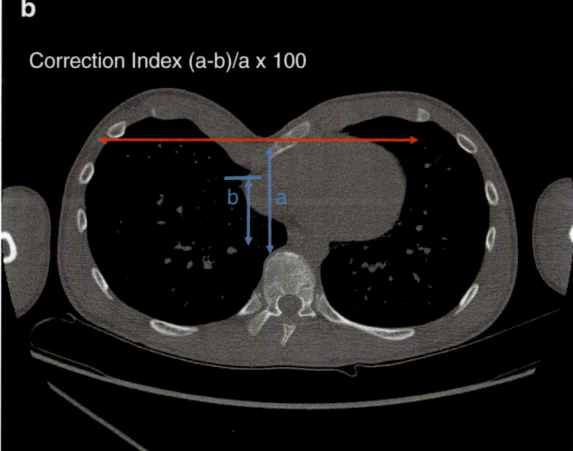

require psychological or psychiatric support prior to consideration of correction where there are worrying signs of anxiety, depression, or body dysmorphia.

7.3.3   Functional Impairment

Compression of intrathoracic structures secondary to the deformity causes a decrease in intrathoracic volume and can lead to cardiac impingement. It is suggested that symptoms may worsen with age, and patients with pectus excavatum have a shorter life expectancy than the general population [1].

The significance of the functional or physical effects of pectus excavatum is controversial and remains an important topic of debate.

7.3.3.1 Pulmonary Function

Pulmonary function tests (PFTs) are regularly performed to investigate exertional breathlessness, 'wheeziness' or associated respiratory problems in patients with pectus deformity. However, they are often difficult to interpret and can appear normal or 'near normal'. More recent reports have sought to clarify the type of testing, what is 'normal' in a usual healthy young group of individuals within a Gaussian (bell curve) model and the degree of severity of the pectus excavatum. Kelly and colleagues in a large series of patients with severe pectus excavatum demonstrated that, when considered against findings in a normal population with PFT values distributed according to a Gaussian (bell curve) and 100% predicted is under the centre of that curve, the bell curve of FVC, FEV1 and FEV 25–75 is shifted to significantly lower values in pectus excavatum [4].

It appears that patients with severe pectus excavatum (Haller index >7, with normal index 2.2 and severe pectus excavatum >3.25) were much more likely to have restrictive PFTs (defined as FVC <80% predicted, with a normal ratio of FEV1 to FVC) than those with a Haller index of <7 [4, 5].

Attention more recently has turned to possible mechanisms of lung dysfunction, particularly the role of chest wall movement and its effects as studied using 3D topographical imaging and oculo electronic plethysmography (OEP) [5]. The relationship of very severe deformity and restrictive PFTs coupled with OEP measurements demonstrating very deep depressions that have the greatest volume fixed incursion into the bony thorax has been described [5].

Though with more defined investigative tools and clearer understanding of variations in lung function across population groups, evidence is emerging that pectus excavatum has an effect; however, controversy still remains on the influence of the pectus severity, the type of corrective surgery and its effectiveness in improving or reversing breathlessness and/or abnormal PFTs after surgical correction before or after the bar is removed [6].

7.3.3.2 Cardiac Function

The effect of sternal displacement posteriorly particularly in severe pectus excavatum is obvious radiologically and echocardiographically and causes cardiac compression, with an anterior indentation of the right ventricle. Early studies suggested a functional effect on the heart, typically with the left ventricular end-diastolic volume index and stroke volume index increased at rest after surgical correction [6]. However, despite these early studies, no consensus has been reached on the significance of cardiac and cardiopulmonary dysfunction and pectus excavatum [6, 7] (Fig. 7.2).

A recent review including studies that examined cardiac output and exercise capacity (through cardiopulmonary exercise testing, CPET, or VO_2 max) concluded that measures of cardiac output such as stroke volume during exercise generally increased regardless of the type of corrective surgery though it was not significant in all studies. It postulated that this was due to the relief of compressed cardiac chambers and overall improved filling of the heart. In addition, though not all studies demonstrated an improvement, overall more studies than not showed an increase in exercise capacity following surgical correction regardless of the type of operation. However, some limitations in the studies were highlighted including number, age and endpoints measured [7].

7.4   Pre-operative Assessment

Clinical assessment of patients with pectus excavatum should include their height, weight and chest wall measurements ideally including photography and 3D body scan. Assessment of the suppleness of the deformity can be performed by observing the degree of correction of the deformity when the patient performs a Valsalva manoeuvre, that is, by attempting to forcibly exhale whilst keeping the mouth and nose closed. By increasing the intrathoracic pressure during the manoeuvre, the flexible anterior chest wall and sternum are driven forward, autocorrecting the excavatum (Table 7.2).

Fig. 7.2 MRI showing significant cardiac compression

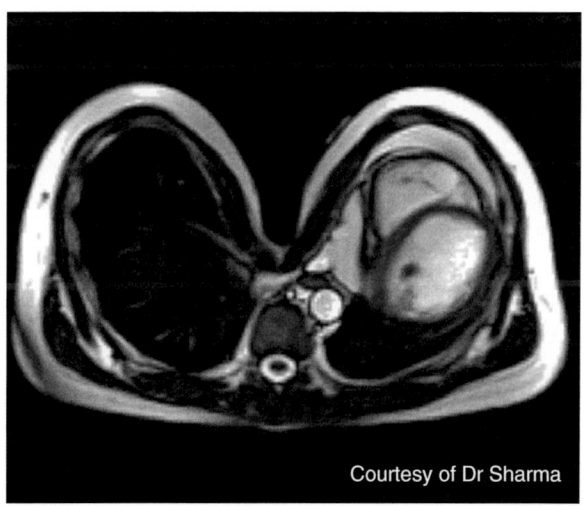

Courtesy of Dr Sharma

Table 7.2 Alongside clinical examination, the pre-assessment for corrective pectus surgery includes

Indication	Investigation
All	Chest wall measurements, medical photography and/or 3D body scan
	Chest CT or MRI to assess severity and associated features such as sternal rotation as well as calculation of HI and CI
In the presence of symptoms:	
Breathlessness	Lung function tests. Consider CPET
Palpitations, syncope or pre-syncope	ECG, transthoracic echocardiogram. Consider stress echocardiogram
Significant psychological features	Psychological assessment
Features of Marfan syndrome	Chest CT, transthoracic echocardiogram, genetic referral for fibrillin-1 mutation and ophthalmology review
Those undergoing bar insertion including the Nuss procedure	Metal allergy testing (titanium bars can be considered if there is a metal allergy)

7.5   Operative Techniques

The two most common types of corrective surgical repair of pectus excavatum are the 'open' modified Ravitch operation and MIRPE (minimally invasive repair of pectus excavatum) or the Nuss procedure. The choice of procedure depends on factors including age of patient, severity of deformity, associated significant asymmetry and sternal rotation, risk of complications and the experience of the surgical team.

A recent systematic review and meta-analysis of the Ravitch and Nuss procedures for pectus excavatum extending to both paediatric and adult patient groups noted no significant difference between the open versus the minimally invasive patients in terms of age, gender (majority male) and CT chest index. The operation duration was significantly shorter for the Nuss procedure, though hospital stay was comparable. Parameters such as post-operative pain, analgesia duration and operative blood loss could not be pooled. Though the review noted many limitations in analysing the current literature, not least the variability of surgical technique employed, it concluded that no differences were noted in the Nuss and Ravitch procedures for paediatric patients, but in adults the Ravitch appeared to result in fewer complications [8].

7.5.1   Open Repair of Pectus Excavatum

7.5.1.1 Ravitch Procedure
Published in 1949 by Dr. Mark Ravitch, the paper described a midline incision in children, elevation of the pectoral muscles bilaterally and resection of the costal cartilages together with the perichondrium. Each deformed costal cartilage segment

was completely resected from sternum to costochondral junction. In addition, Ravitch described dividing xiphisternal articulation [or junction] and substernal ligament and resecting the associated costal cartilages. A transverse osteotomy at the sterno-manubrial junction was then performed and essentially fractured the sternum at this point and held in place using sutures. No attempt was made to suture the remaining cartilage ends [chondral ends of the ribs] to the sternum as the defect was too extensive. No sternal support was used.

Ravitch described how typically the lower 3–5 costal cartilages were resected bilaterally and to their fullest extent (with presumed preservation of the manubrium and its costal connections).

Note the Ravitch and subsequent modifications of the original operation can also surgically correct pectus carinatum deformities.

7.5.1.2 Modified Ravitch Procedure

The 'modified' Ravitch procedure was first attributed to Ravitch in 1965 [9]. Modifications from the original Ravitch procedure most noticeably include subperichondrial excision of variable lengths of the costal cartilage preserving much of the perichondrium sheath (the connective tissue layer that envelops cartilage), partial and if necessary multiple wedge osteotomies with or without internal fixation and lifting the sternum using internal supports (usually metal bars) to 'hold' the sternum forward. At present, most patients undergo a modified version of this procedure as described below.

Modified Ravitch involves a general anaesthetic in the supine position. Whilst double-lumen intubation may be useful, it is not essential. Patients may be given the choice of a vertical midline (Fig. 7.3) or transverse inframammary incision (often

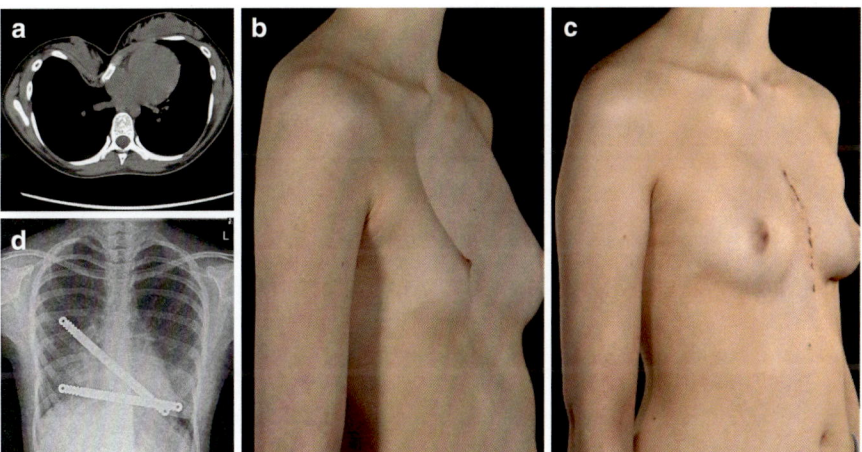

Fig. 7.3 (**a**) Pre-operative chest CT demonstrating severe and asymmetric deformity. (**b**) Preoperative photos before and (**c**) 2 weeks following modified Ravitch procedure. (**d**) Post-operative chest X-ray showing a 2-bar internal support using a partial 'cross-bar' method to maximise correction

Fig. 7.4 Intraoperative
photo of a submammary
approach (looking toward
the head) and modified
Ravitch procedure using
two Marlex mesh
'hammocks', avoiding a
second procedure to
remove metal supports

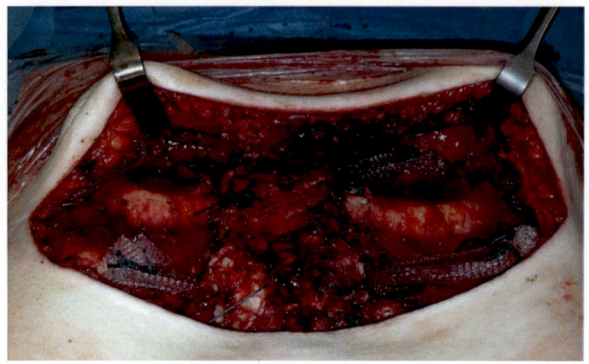

offered in females) (Fig. 7.4). However, patients with a high deformity may require a vertical incision to access the costal cartilage above the fourth rib. The medial aspects of pectoralis major muscles are dissected from the sternum and elevated as a flap up until the lateral edge of the costal cartilage and the highest costal cartilage involved in the deformity is accessible. The abdominal muscles are mobilised inferiorly just enough to expose the lower deformed cartilages. Each abnormal costal cartilage involved in the deformity is then resected from the bony edge of the anterior rib to the sternum. The periosteum is first incised with a scalpel or cautery and the cartilage cut at each end. The cartilage is bluntly dissected from the inferior periosteum and removed with bone holding forceps, preserving the perichondrial sheath and care taken to avoid injury to the associated neurovascular bundle laterally and the mammary vessels medially. The extent of cartilage resection is variable with some surgeons performing total cartilage resection as described by Ravitch, whilst others remove only minimal cartilage to allow disarticulation from the sternum [10]. If less cartilage is excised, the perichondrial sheaths are usually re-approximated to the sternum using absorbable sutures. Once the abnormal cartilages are excised bilaterally, a saw can be used to perform one or more sternal wedge-shaped osteotomy where there is significant sternal angulation or rotation. Typically, the osteotomy is partial, preserving the posterior periosteal table and allowing for correction of sternal rotation in asymmetric pectus excavatum. This can then be sutured to support the elevation. The xiphoid is freed from the sternum through a transverse incision if required, and then sutured back to the sternum. Several different materials can then be used to elevate the sternum based on the surgeon or patient's preference. Usually a metal bar is used and secured, but would require a second operation to remove. Therefore, alternative materials have included Marlex mesh 'sling or hammock' which is sutured or secured onto the ribs on each side [11]. Once careful haemostasis has been undertaken, the wounds are closed in layers with the pectoralis muscles approximated in the midline and a subcutaneous drain inserted to avoid formation of a haematoma. Some surgeons advocate actively draining the pleural space.

7.5.2 Nuss Procedure

There are now many years of data regarding this procedure since it was first described in 1987 by Dr. Donald Nuss, and it is the most common procedure performed for pectus excavatum correction. Since that first report, there have been many modifications to this minimally invasive pectus excavatum repair [12], but the technique fundamentally remains unchanged, that is, the placement of an internal 'brace' to lift the sternum without excision of the cartilage.

The procedure involves a general anaesthetic with or without double-lumen intubation depending on age and/or CO_2 insufflation (up to 5–10 mmHg depending on age and size of patient), which is most often used to obtain collapse of the lung. The patient is placed in a supine position. The arms may be tucked in at the sides or placed in a crucifix position or partially abducted depending on the surgeon's preference. Patients are grouped and saved, and a median sternotomy set including a saw is readily available (Fig. 7.5).

Selecting and marking the surgical landmarks for bar position is important. Our practice is to prep the skin and drape the patient, followed by marking and then covering with an incise skin drape (Opsite®). The deepest point of the deformity is marked, followed laterally on either side the sites for entry of the bar into the chest (generally the highest points of the deformity). Finally, a bar template is used to

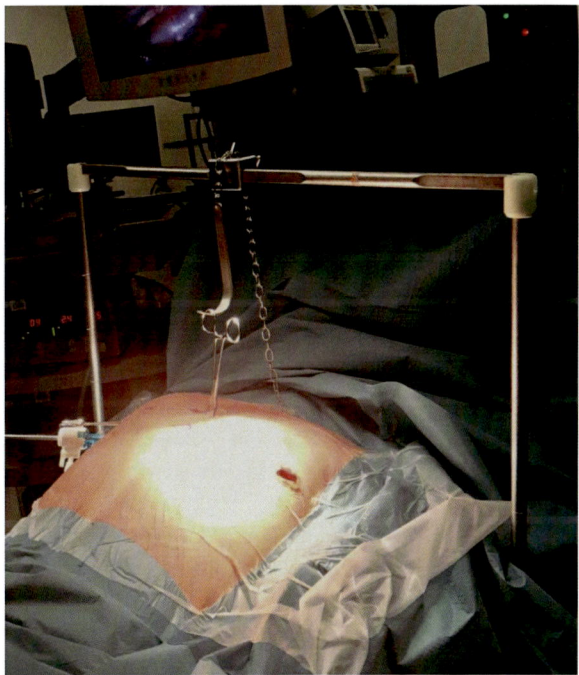

Fig. 7.5 The patient is placed supine with arms tucked and an inflatable bag placed behind the shoulder blades and inflated prior to the procedure. The senior author uses a Gollinger cross-bar type retractor and bone holding forceps to grasp the sternum at the deepest point of depression which is then lifted and the bag deflated

measure the sites of the skin incisions laterally and to decide on the length of bar to be used. There has been a tendency to use shorter bars and place skin incision more anteriorly accordingly rather than at the midaxillary line [13]. Our practice is having measured with the bar template and selected the length of the bar for that patient; the skin incisions are marked in front of the midaxillary line and are marked perpendicular (approximately 3–4 cm). The use of two bars particularly in older patients with asymmetric, wider or deeper deformities or when the deepest point is below or inferior to the sternum has become common [12]. Care is taken to mark both positions of entry into the chest with one bar usually marked as sitting below the deepest point and the second bar under the lower sternum. The two bars can be positioned through one or two skin incisions bilaterally.

The case begins with the insertion of a 5 mm 30° thoracoscope on the right side via a trocar aimed superiorly. Our practice is to utilise the right-sided skin incision for placement of the trocar as low as possible though others including the Nuss place the port separately [12]. Most surgeons insert the scope on the right, though inserting on the left or both sides of the chest are described. Regardless of the side, thoracoscopic visualisation of the deformity is essential for bar placement. Several audio-visual pectus devices have been developed for the sole purpose of safe placement of the bar across the mediastinum including the pectoscope (an adapted combined thoracoscope and introducer) [14]. Following port insertion and CO_2 insufflation, the right pleural cavity and mediastinum are carefully examined, particularly noting if the deepest part of the deformity corresponds to the external markings of the entry sites (Fig. 7.6).

In severe, deep or very asymmetrical deformities, the importance of being able to lift the sternum during the procedure has become increasingly recognised and aids the safety of crossing the pleural cavities with an introducer, avoiding pericardial or even cardiac injury. Various modified or bespoke surgical devices to aid lifting of the sternum have been developed, including retractors such as the Rultract® Skyhook Retractor System, the Crane technique [14] and the vacuum bell method [15].

The method we employ follows a stab incision placed at the deepest point in the midline and/or on the sternal side that is most depressed if the deformity is asymmetric, and the anterior table at the sternal edge is grasped, lifted and suspended off the Gollinger retractor. The inflatable bag is then deflated and the sternum is lifted, allowing a gap to open between the back end of the sternum and the pericardium (Fig. 7.6a, b).

The second contralateral skin incision is made where previously marked at the anterior axillary line and is taken down through the subcutaneous tissues to the ribcage taking care not to divide intercostal muscle.

The subcutaneous tunnels are then created, using a Langenbeck retractor to lift, whilst blunt dissection is completed up to the point marked at the site of entry. A right-angled instrument is used to breach the pleura and enter the chest cavity under direct thoracoscopic vision. The contralateral subcutaneous tunnel is then created to the mark of bar exit and the pleura is again breached using a right-angled instrument. Care is taken when breaching the pleura as the heart can be significantly shifted to the left.

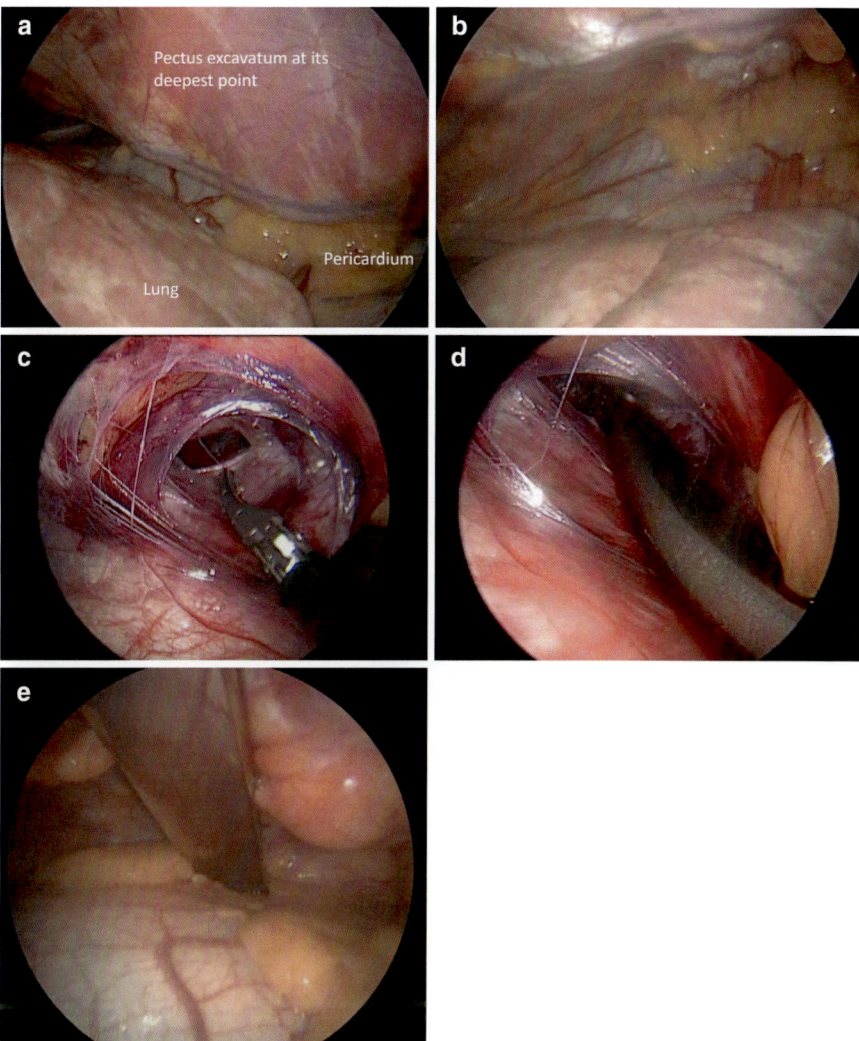

Fig. 7.6 (a–e) Following the preparation of both lateral skin incisions and insertion of the thoracoscope. The deformity is assessed and if necessary the sternum is lifted. Thoracoscopic image looking toward the mediastinum (**a**) before and after lifting the sternum (**b**). The anterior mediastinum is dissected using an endodissector (**c**) dissecting across the contralateral pleural cavity to allow safe passage of the introducer (**d**). The bar is positioned in relation to the deepest point and turned immediately correcting the pectus excavatum (**e**)

Various methods of passing the introducer across the mediastinum have been described, but current convention is that it must be performed under direct vision at all times as risk of serious injury to mediastinal structures is possible at this stage, though the risk is very low [16]. Many surgeons use the introducer itself as the dissector, but it is our practice to formally dissect across the mediastinum using an endoscopic grasper (Maryland®). The endoscopic grasper is inserted through the right skin incision at the most superior point and the pleural reflection at the mediastinum opened under thoracoscopic guidance (Fig. 7.6c). The dissection starts superiorly where the sternum tends to be at the highest point. Once the pleural reflection is breached just below the surface of the sternum, the CO_2 helps the dissection by 'diffusing' through the 'filmy' anterior mediastinal soft tissue as well as reducing capillary bleeding due to the raised intrathoracic pressure. Endoscopic dissection is completely through blunt dissection crossing the mediastinum, taking care to separate the filmy mediastinal connective tissue from the underlying pericardium and overlying under the surface of the sternum. Once the mediastinum is crossed, the contralateral pleural reflection is breached and the endoscopic grasper is seen to enter the contralateral pleural cavity. During endoscopic dissection as well as moving across the mediastinum from right pleural cavity to the left, dissection is carried in a cranial to caudal direction, approaching the deepest point of the deformity.

The curved introducer is now introduced in the pleural cavity through the subcutaneous tunnel and through the entry point with tip pointing down, and then once in, it is turned with tip pointing up and is passed through the dissected mediastinal tissue plane under direct vision and keeping the tip in view as it is passed (Fig. 7.6d). It is helpful for ECG monitoring with an 'audible' signal and anaesthetic team to be aware to monitor for cardiac arrhythmias during the insertion of the introducer. Once passed to the mediastinum, the handle of the introducer often has to be pushed down, pointing the curved toward the contralateral anterior chest wall, and this can be aided by having a finger inserted through the exit site to guide the tip through. Very occasionally, particularly in very deep and symmetrical deformities, if the tip is not immediately felt and the introducer guided out through the bar exit site, it is very simple to either cross the mediastinum with the thoracoscope or even insert the thoracoscope through the contralateral skin incision and allow direct visualisation of the tip to help guide it through the bar exit site. Once the introducer is pushed through the exit site in the corresponding intercostal space on the left side, care is taken not to 'strip' the intercostal muscle off the rib interspace, by lifting up on the introducer tip as it passes through the subcutaneous tunnel whilst simultaneously pressing across the interspace 'guarding' the intercostal muscles.

Once the introducer has been pulled through, it is left in position elevating the sternum whilst the bar is prepared. The introducer can be lifted bilaterally in preparation for bar insertion to allow chest wall tissues to stretch and the tension on the introducer to become less. There is also an opportunity to check the position of the introducer thoracoscopically, the need for a second bar, as well as check for acceptable clearance from the pericardium.

Using the bar template, the bar is prepared by bending to confirm the shape of the patient's chest. Using a tape or a 28 Fr chest drain securely sutured to the introducer tip, the introducer is removed carefully under thoracoscopic guidance, and the bar is then attached to the tape or sutured to the drain tip on the left side and pulled across the mediastinum to the right side of the chest. This is done with the bar convexity facing the patient's mediastinum, and once it has entered the pleural cavity, it is carefully turned and passed across the chest under thoracoscopic guidance as the attached tape or drain is removed. Once in a satisfactory position with the tips of the bar exiting the skin incisions of either side, bar flippers are attached to each side and the bar is inverted into a concave position. This can be done either as a clockwise or anticlockwise manoeuvre depending on the deepest point of the deformity. The bar should sit on the ribcage comfortably without being too tight (Fig. 7.7a–d). Occasionally, reversing the flipping and even the insertion process is required and the bar needs to be re-fashioned. The bar can then be secured on either or both sides with a stabiliser. This is essential to avoid bar displacement. There has been a tendency to use only one stabiliser as bar removal is easier and that is very acceptable. The stabiliser has to be positioned medially to provide support and reduce the risk of the bar displacing. The stabiliser is then secured to the underlying soft tissues and rib using a heavy PDS suture.

To avoid insertion of an intercostal chest drain, a small-bore suction catheter can be inserted through the 5 mm camera port with the other end placed into a small pot of water, creating an underwater seal as the lung is re-inflated. The catheter is positioned toward the top of the pleural cavity, the patient is placed into a reverse Trendelenburg position (head up), and the lung is inflated either passively or with the help of the anaesthetist performing a Valsalva manoeuvre to ensure that there is no residual pneumothorax. If there is no persistent bubbling, the catheter is removed and the wounds are closed in layers with dissolvable sutures such as Vicryl and Monocryl. A chest X-ray is performed in the recovery area to check for a residual pneumothorax.

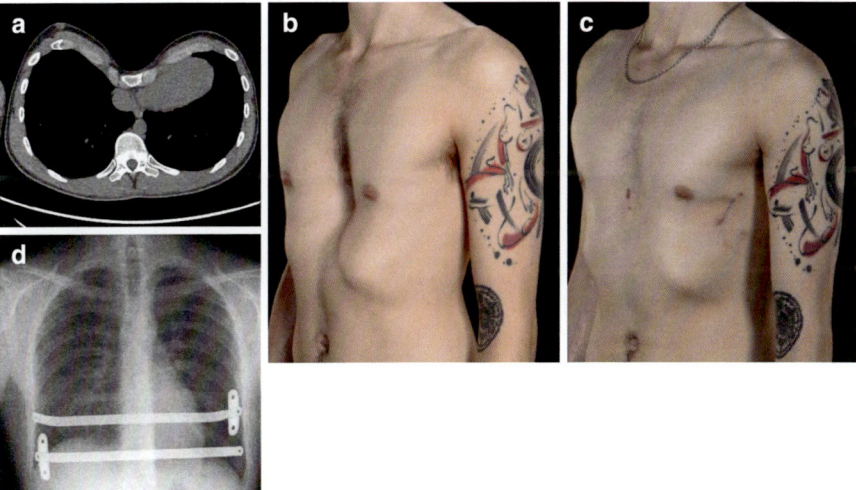

Fig. 7.7 (**a**) Pre-operative chest CT demonstrating severe and asymmetric deformity. (**b**) Pre-operative photos before and (**c**) 2 weeks following a Nuss procedure. (**d**) Post-operative chest X-ray showing a 2-bar technique with one stabiliser on each bar

7.5.3 Variations

Recently several innovative adjuncts to the Nuss procedure have been published, particularly in dealing with more challenging cases. Dr. Hyung Joo Park has described several techniques in managing patients with more complex, deep or eccentric pectus excavatum (often described as a Grand Canyon deformity) including a cross-bar technique [14], as well as 'sandwich technique' developed for managing complex mixed deformities [16].

7.6 Post-operative Care

An enhanced recovery format may be advised in the peri-operative period, focusing on minimising the period of starvation and mobilising the patients early in their recovery. Essential to this is good peri- and post-operative analgesia. A combination of oral and IV analgesia alongside an epidural is often beneficial, particularly in patients undergoing a Nuss procedure. A recent review found that epidural analgesia may provide superior pain control but was comparable with PCA for secondary outcomes [17]. Our practice is to use bilateral intercostal blocks, PCA and a pain protocol-based oral NSAIDs in the immediate post-operative period. Additional physiotherapy including incentive spirometry is recommended. Patients are hospitalised until mobilising comfortably with an average length of stay of 3–4 days post-operatively.

7.7 Bar Removal

Removing the bar is universally recommended but does not always happen. The bar and/or bars are usually removed 2–3 years after insertion, depending on factors such as age at insertion. Removal requires a general anaesthetic and re-opening one or both of the previous lateral incisions. The bar is dissected out of the soft tissues which sometimes can form a bony callus that needs to be removed and can increase the amount of dissection required. The bar is bent so that it passes through the chest smoothly. If two stabilisers have been used, one of them needs to be detached from the bar prior to removal. Typically, the procedure requires an overnight stay in the hospital and occasionally when soft tissue drains are required longer if dissection of the bar from the chest wall is significant. Increasingly, due to reported complications of bar removal [18, 19], full preparation for thoracoscopic assessment and chest opening should be considered.

7.8 Complications

Generally, it appears the risks of the modified Ravitch and Nuss procedures are similar, though certainly very serious complications including death from cardiac or great vessel injury are reported more frequently following Nuss procedures [18] (Table 7.3). The incidence of complications varies from 2 to 20%. The most severe

Table 7.3 Early (A) and late complications (B) following Nuss procedures (based on [12])

(A) Early complications	(B) Late complications
Pneumothorax requiring chest drain	Bar displacement requiring revision
Pleural effusion requiring drainage	Wound issues including seroma, dehiscence, late infection
Haemothorax	Bar allergy
Wound site infection	Overcorrection
Pericarditis	Recurrence
Temporary paralysis	
Cardiac injury including perforation	Haemorrhage with bar removal
Other major vascular injuries including injury to IMA	
Death	

complications of surgery include death or a cardiac event, typically relating to a cardiac arrhythmia or severe anaphylaxis [17, 18]. Patients should also be counselled about the possibility of bleeding, unilateral or bilateral intercostal chest drains for pneumothoraces or pleural collections and of complications relating to the metalwork including bar displacement. Finally, infection, wound problems and recurrence of deformity can also occur in the post-operative period. The modified Ravitch procedure may also be associated with long-term chest wall instability and/or pain.

7.9   Conclusions

Surgical correction of pectus excavatum should be tailored to the individual based on the severity of the deformity, careful evaluation of symptoms and patient choice. Intervention in childhood is associated with fewer complications than older patients; however, care is required in this young and often vulnerable patient population. Both minimally invasive and open procedures have been demonstrated to be safe and efficacious.

References

1. Kragten HA, Siebenga J, Höppener PF, Verburg R, Visker N. Symptomatic pectus excavatum in seniors (SPES): a cardiovascular problem?: a prospective cardiological study of 42 seniors with a symptomatic pectus excavatum. Neth Heart J. 2011;19:73–8.
2. Luo L, Xu B, Wang X, Tan B, Zhao J. Intervention of the Nuss procedure on the mental health of pectus excavatum patients. Ann Thorac Cardiovasc Surg. 2017;23(4):175–80. https://doi.org/10.5761/atcs.oa.17-00014.
3. Poston PM, Patel SS, Rajput M, Rossi NO, Ghanamah MS, Davis JE, Turek JW. The correction index: setting the standard for recommending operative repair of pectus excavatum. Ann Thorac Surg. 2014;97(4):1176–9; discussion 1179–80.
4. Lawson ML, Mellins RB, Paulson JF, Shamberger RC, Oldham K, Azizkhan RG, Hebra AV, Nuss D, Goretsky MJ, Sharp RJ, Holcomb GW III, Shim WK, Megison SM, Moss RL, Fecteau AH, Colombani PM, Moskowitz AB, Hill J, Kelly RE Jr. Increasing severity of pectus excavatum is associated with reduced pulmonary function. J Pediatr. 2011;159(2):256–61.e2.

5. Kelly RE Jr, Obermeyer RJ, Nuss D. Diminished pulmonary function in pectus excavatum: from denying the problem to finding the mechanism. Ann Cardiothorac Surg. 2016;5(5):466–75.
6. Jayaramakrishnan K, Wotton R, Bradley A, Naidu B. Does repair of pectus excavatum improve cardiopulmonary function? Interact Cardiovasc Thorac Surg. 2013;16(6):865–70.
7. Maagaard M, Heiberg J. Improved cardiac function and exercise capacity following correction of pectus excavatum: a review of current literature. Ann Cardiothorac Surg. 2016;5(5):485–92.
8. Kanagaratnam A, Phan S, Tchantchaleishvilli V, Phan K. Ravitch versus Nuss procedure for pectus excavatum: systematic review and meta-analysis. Ann Cardiothoracic Surg. 2016;5(5):409–21.
9. Ravitch MM. Technical problems in the operative correction of pectus excavatum. Ann Surg. 1965;162:29–33.
10. Fonkalsrud EW. Open repair of pectus excavatum with minimal cartilage resection. Ann Surg. 2004;240(2):231–5.
11. Robicsek F. Marlex mesh support for the correction of very severe and recurrent pectus excavatum. Ann Thorac Surg. 1978;26(1):80–3.
12. Nuss D, Kelly JE. The minimally invasive repair of pectus excavatum. Oper Tech Thorac Cardiovasc Surg. 2014;19(3):324–47.
13. Pilegaard HK. Single centre experience on short bar technique for pectus excavatum. Ann Cardiothorac Surg. 2016;5(5):450–5.
14. Park HJ. A technique for complex pectus excavatum repair: the cross-bar technique for Grand Canyon type deformity (Park classification). Ann Cardiothorac Surg. 2016;5(5):526–7.
15. Schier F, Bahr M, Klobe E. The vacuum chest wall lifter: an innovative, nonsurgical addition to the management of pectus excavatum. J Pediatr Surg. 2005;40(3):496–500.
16. Park HJ, Kim KS. The sandwich technique for repair of pectus carinatum and excavatum/carinatum complex. Ann Cardiothorac Surg. 2016;5(5):434–9.
17. Frawley G, Frawley J, Crameri J. A review of anesthetic techniques and outcomes following minimally invasive repair of pectus excavatum (Nuss procedure). Paediatr Anaesth. 2016;26(11):1082–90.
18. Hebra A, Kelly RE, Ferro MM, Yüksel M, Campos JRM, Nuss D. Life-threatening complications and mortality of minimally invasive pectus surgery. J Pediatr Surg. 2018;53(4):728–32. pii: S0022–3468(17)30461-X.
19. Park HJ, Kim KS. Pectus bar removal: surgical technique and strategy to avoid complications. J Vis Surg. 2016;2:60.

Pectus Excavatum: Functional Respiratory Impact, Quality of Life, and Preoperative Assessment

Louis Daussy, Elise Noel-Savina, Alain Didier, and Daniel Riviere

8.1   Introduction

Pectum excavatum's (PE) functional impact is discussed. To this day, there is no consensus despite the many studies published on that subject. This explains that there are no official guidelines regarding the evaluation of patients with PE. However, some authors suggested guidelines on the indications of corrective surgery (Nuss, or modified Ravitch) [1–3]. But the definition of functional respiratory and cardiac impairment may not be described precisely enough. Moreover, they used a radiological measure (Haller index) although several studies showed a lack of correlation with the physiological impairment of the deformity [4–6] and no impact on the patient's quality of life [7, 8]. The aesthetic damage and its psycho-social impact were not always considered. The plastic surgery solutions were not part of the decision algorithm.

Surgical techniques correcting the deformity are associated with significant post-operative pain and complications, whose frequency and potential severity, may lead the reconsider their benefit-risk ratio. This is especially true since the development of less invasive plastic techniques that can offer a convincing aesthetic solution.

In this chapter, we tried to make a state of knowledge about the impact of PE, both on the physiology and on the health-related quality of life. As explained previously,

L. Daussy (✉)
Pulmonary Department, Albi Hospital, Albi, France
e-mail: louis.daussy@ch-albi.fr

E. Noel-Savina · D. Riviere
Pulmonary Department, Larrey Hospital, Toulouse University Hospital, Toulouse, France
e-mail: noel-savina.e@chu-toulouse.fr; riviere.d@chu-toulouse.fr

A. Didier
Pulmunology and Allergology Department, Larrey Hospital, Toulouse University Hospital, Toulouse, France
e-mail: didier.a@chu-toulouse.fr

© Springer Nature Switzerland AG 2019
J.-P. Chavoin (ed.), *Pectus Excavatum and Poland Syndrome Surgery*,
https://doi.org/10.1007/978-3-030-05108-2_8

because there are no official guidelines, we suggested an evaluation strategy for these patients. We also described the surgical solutions that seemed to have the best benefit-risk ratio in each situation, including plastic surgical techniques.

On several occasions, we quoted the results of a study by Dupuis et al. which is not yet published. It focused on the preoperative evaluation of 60 PE patients before plastic surgery using the technique of Prof. Chavoin [9]. The studied parameters were respiratory function, exercise abilities, and quality of life.

8.2   Pectus Excavatum and Symptoms

To this day, there is no consensus on whether PE causes symptoms. While some patients with PE may have no complaints, symptoms are described in the literature and their prevalence varies widely depending on the studies. This variability is probably related to differences in the way of collecting information but also to different recruitment methods that can generate selection bias on clinical severity. In the work of Dupuis et al., where the mean Haller index was similar to the one in other cohorts of patients who underwent corrective surgery [9–11], 93% of the patients were asymptomatic. In other studies, up to 80% of patients had an exercise intolerance [7, 12], 70% an exertional dyspnoea [4, 7, 12], 67% had episodes of chest tightness [4, 7, 12], and 51% experienced chest pain [3–5]. However, in none of these studies there is a control group to prove that the prevalence of these symptoms was greater than in the general population.

Some studies describe, after corrective surgery, an improvement and sometimes a disappearance of complaints that may concern up to 96% of initially symptomatic patients [13, 14].

8.3   Pectus and Functional Impairment

8.3.1   Respiratory Function at Rest

The consequences of PE on respiratory function is a long-standing question in the literature. Although many studies describe the respiratory function of patients with PE, the differences in the study designs, in the age of patients and in the definition of a functional impact make it difficult to answer this question. The response mostly depends on the definition of a ventilatory impairment.

PE patients appear to have some ventilatory parameters below the expected values. A publication on a large cohort, found that the distribution of values of the vital capacity (VC) or the forced expiratory volume in one second (FEV1) in these patients, took the aspect of Gaussian curves whose peaks were at 88% and 83%, respectively, and not 100% as in the general population [15].

The impairment can also be defined by a ventilatory function out of the normal range. Most of the time results are expressed in average +/− standard deviation and only a few studies describe the prevalence of ventilatory disorders in cohorts of patients with a PE. In this case, it is most often a small cohort, and the definition of ventilatory disorders can differ from one study to another, or is not specified.

The prevalence of obstructive airway disorders in PE patients ranges from 5% to 42% depending on the definition and the population studied [4, 16, 17]. However, the high prevalence of confounding comorbidities such as asthma in these makes it difficult to draw conclusions about the accountability of PE in these disorders. In addition, the lack of correlation between the severity of the deformity, defined by a high Haller index, and parameters that classically evaluate obstructive respiratory disease (FEV1, FEV1/FVC, and DEM25-75) reduces the accountability of PE in these obstructive disorders [18].

In most studies, mean total lung capacity (TLC) and vital capacity (VC) are within the normal range if defined by a value greater than or equal to 80% of the predicted value (pv) [12, 19]. In the few studies that described the prevalence of restrictive disorders using TLC, it varies from 0% in the study of Dupuis et al. [9] to 6% [4, 16]. It seems, however, that PE is more likely to affect mobilizable volumes than total lung volume, as suggested by a study showing a decreased CV (<80% of pv) in 25% of patients with PE [12]. However, to this day, decreased VC with normal TLC is not considered a ventilatory disorder [20].

Patients with PE do not seem to have impaired exercise ventilatory functions based on current literature data. Indeed, several studies found that the mean ventilatory reserve, during VO_2 max tests, was within the limits of normal [4, 21] or was not different from the mean values of a control group [22]. Some studies suggested a variation of some ventilatory features during exercise such as a slight limitation in the increase of tidal volume compensated by a greater rise in the respiratory rate [4]. But it was not considered as pathological because the ventilatory reserve was normal. Dupuis et al. found only two cases, out of 60 patients, of ventilatory limitation for which the accountability of the PE could not be excluded.

8.3.2 Cardiac Function

Studies showed improvements in some morphological parameters of the right heart cavities after corrective surgery, indicating compression by the sternum [23–25]. Moreover, the prevalence of valvular diseases such as mitral valve prolapse associated or not with mitral insufficiency is increased and may concern up to 50% of patients compared to 8% in a control group [25, 26].

Regarding the cardiac output, it does not seem altered at rest [27] but several studies suggested repercussions during exercise. Some publications found a lower ability to increase the volume of systolic ejection (VES) during incremental exercises. Although this is compensated by heart rate, when it reaches its maximum value above a certain intensity, the ability to increase the cardiac output is limited [5, 28] .

8.3.3 Evolution of Functional Parameters after Surgery Correcting the Thoracic Deformity

Data is not in favour of a clinically relevant improvement of the ventilatory function at rest. There is a gain of only a few percent of the mean values of VC, TLC, and FEV1, expressed as a percentage of predicted value, even though they are already within normal limits before surgery [19]. Regarding the ventilatory parameters during exercise, the results after surgery are discordant but, overall, do not find a clinically relevant evolution [10, 23, 29].

Valvular diseases do not systematically improve after surgery. This suggests that the compression by sternal depression might not be the only aetiology. The mitral valve prolapse is corrected in only 20–40% of cases and mitral insufficiency doesn't disappear but improves in nearly half of the cases [25, 26]. Regarding cardiac output during exercise, a 2013 publication on children and adolescents showed a lower preoperative cardiac index than in the control group, whereas in the re-evaluation 3 years after Nuss surgery, this difference disappeared, suggesting a normalization of cardiac function during exercise [5]. However, a similar study with a small cohort of adults did not find any improvement 1 year after Nuss surgery [30].

The results regarding the evolution of the exercise abilities are discordant. While some publications do not find a post-operative improvement of the mean VO_2 max [5, 11, 27, 29–31], others find an improvement that remains modest and of questionable clinical relevance [10, 32–35].

Thus, the impact of PE on ventilatory function is rare, and the main problem seems to be the cardiac function during exercise. However, regarding exercise abilities, the benefit of corrective surgery does not seem obvious. It seems to improve patients with symptoms.

Nevertheless, further studies on large cohorts are necessary to improve our knowledge about the cardiac exercise impact of PE, to specify its prevalence, and to define a "cut off" of clinical relevance. More works are necessary to define which patients could have a relevant functional benefit from corrective surgeries. Given the current data, the functional benefit of these surgeries appears to be modest and could make us reconsider the benefit-risk ratio given the complications they can cause. It might be interesting to focus on patients with preoperative respiratory or cardiac repercussions.

8.3.4 Pectus Excavatum and Quality of Life

Chest deformity can impair the quality of life and its correction by conventional surgical techniques (Ravitch, Nuss) can improve it. Since the advent of plastic surgery, it seems important now to try to distinguish what influences this improvement, the correction of the aesthetic problem, or a possible functional impact. Publications using quality-of-life questionnaires have found an alteration in "physical functioning" score [36] compared to a control population. Others described improvements in "physical stamina" scores [37] or "physical difficulties" [8] after corrective surgery. In contrast, Dupuis et al. [9] found no decrease in "physical functioning" and "role physical" scores in their cohort of patients compared to the values of the general population of the same age and sex. The data is discordant on the consequences on quality of life of the functional repercussions of PE; but the impact of aesthetic damage on quality of life is less debated. The deformity can alter patients' body image and impair their self-esteem, which can have important repercussions on their psychological and social functioning. It can lead up to anxio-depressive disorders or withdrawal behaviour [38]. Corrective surgeries significantly improve the psycho-social functioning of these patients [8, 36, 37], but similar results were found after plastic surgery correcting only the aesthetics [39].

This suggests that the aesthetic problem is the main, and sometimes the only, cause of the alteration of quality of life. It is well illustrated by the fact that the aesthetic complaint is by far the most frequent request for surgery, and when associated with a functional complaint, it is most of the time the main motive [40].

8.4   The Assessment of Patients with PE

Interrogation and clinical examination must be rigorous and have two main objectives:

– To scan for elements pointing to a syndromic form of PE such as Marfan's disease. The situations requiring a consultation with a geneticist in a patient with a PE have been described by Cobben et al. [41].
– To focus on whether patients experience symptoms such as dyspnoea, exercise intolerance, palpitation, chest pain, or tightness. If so, it is important to clarify when they have appeared, whether they tend to worsen over time, their severity and if they are perceived as disabling in everyday life.

It is important to evaluate PE patients with the following tests:

– A functional respiratory test (body plethysmography) should be performed, looking for a restrictive syndrome. Its current definition is a CPT lower than the value corresponding to the fifth percentile, or with a Z-score < −1.64. If an obstructive ventilatory disorder is identified, it is first necessary to search for another aetiology then the PE such as asthma and therefore a bronchodilator reversibility test must be performed. An obstructive pattern is defined by a FEV1/VC under the value corresponding to the fifth percentile (Z-score < 1.64), except when other comorbidities with a specific cutoff are suspected, such as chronic obstructive pulmonary disease (COPD) (FEV1/CV < 0.7) [42] or asthma (FEV1/CV < 0.75 in adults, <0.9 in children) [20, 42, 43].
– A transthoracic echocardiogram at rest may be useful to search for signs of Marfan's disease (aortic dilation +/− with aortic insufficiency) that could lead to specific treatments and follow-up. It can also detect mitral valvular disease (prolapse +/− associated with mitral insufficiency) or signs of compression of the

right heart cavities, but clinically relevant criteria that would suggest a functional benefit of corrective surgery have not been clearly described yet.

- Thoracic imaging by radiography or thoracic CT is often realized to perform measurements and calculate radiological indices of severity. For Professor Chavoin's technique, it will also allow the modelling of the custom-made silicone implant, thanks to 3D reconstructions.
- A cardiopulmonary exercise test (CPET) with VO_2 max measurement is essential to evaluate the patient's physical abilities and to look for cardiovascular and/or ventilatory limitations during exercise. Abnormally low physical abilities that are not explained by physical deconditioning are in favour of a functional impact of PE on exercise, even more if there are signs of functional limitation. The limitation can be ventilatory, when the ventilatory reserve is decreased whereas there is no sign of over-ventilation. It can be a respiratory limitation if the oxygen saturation decreases during exercise. As there is no measurement of functional cardiac parameters during CPET except for blood pressure, this test can only suggest a cardiovascular limitation but cannot formally prove it. It is suggested for example, by an abnormally low O_2 pulse at maximal exercise intensity or a hyperkinetic cardiac response that isn't clearly linked with physical deconditioning. In that case, the cardiovascular limitation should ideally be confirmed by assessing the cardiac function at exercise, for example, with a stress echocardiography or a non-invasive measure of cardiac output (PHYSIOFLOW). These tests are not yet performed routinely in this indication.

8.5   Conclusion

The main complaint of patients with PE seems to be aesthetic and can cause psychosocial suffering. This alone can justify surgical management. To this day there is no evidence that the lack of surgical correction of the deformity compromises life expectancy [44]. For this reason, the objective is to offer the solution that best meets the patient's expectations with a minimum risk.

Thus, when a patient requests a surgical treatment of his PE for aesthetic reasons, there are three situations:

- If the patient is asymptomatic and the functional assessment is normal, the benefit/risk balance clearly supports plastic surgeries because they offer good aesthetic results, really low post-operative pain and extremely rare significant complication [39].
- If the patient suffers from a disabling symptomatology suggesting a physical impact of his PE and that its accountability is supported by the presence of significant abnormalities on the functional assessment, it seems reasonable to discuss surgeries correcting osteochondral deformity (modified Ravitch, Nuss). Indeed, these techniques offer both an aesthetic solution and the possibility of improving the symptomatology. Nevertheless, the patient must clearly be

informed of the post-operative pain and the complications related to these surgeries. If he finds them unacceptable or excessive regarding his symptoms, a plastic surgery seems to be a better solution.

– If the patient is asymptomatic but has abnormal functional tests, it is necessary to search further for functional impact. Indeed, it can be hidden by an adaptation of the lifestyle, for example, by avoiding situations that may generate symptoms, such as physical activities. If they have no symptoms, plastic surgery seems to be the best solution. Otherwise both strategies should be discussed, describing their risks and benefits, including the possibility of improving the patient's "neglected symptoms". The patient can then choose the strategy that best suits his current or desired lifestyle.

References

1. Frantz FW. Indications and guidelines for pectus excavatum repair. Curr Opin Pediatr. 2011;23(4):486–91.
2. Nuss D, Kelly RE. Indications and technique of Nuss procedure for pectus excavatum. Thorac Surg Clin. 2010;20(4):583–97.
3. Jaroszewski D, Notrica D, McMahon L, Steidley DE, Deschamps C. Current management of pectus excavatum: a review and update of therapy and treatment recommendations. J Am Board Fam Med. 2010;23(2):230–9.
4. Cavestri B, Wurtz A, Bart F, Nevière R, Aguilaniu B, Wallaert B. [Cardiopulmonary exercise testing in patients with pectus excavatum]. Rev Mal Respir. 2010;27(7):717–23.
5. Maagaard M, Tang M, Ringgaard S, Nielsen HHM, Frøkiær J, Haubuf M, et al. Normalized cardiopulmonary exercise function in patients with pectus excavatum three years after operation. Ann Thorac Surg. 2013;96(1):272–8.
6. Chao C-J, Jaroszewski DE, Kumar PN, Ewais MM, Appleton CP, Mookadam F, et al. Surgical repair of pectus excavatum relieves right heart chamber compression and improves cardiac output in adult patients—an intraoperative transesophageal echocardiographic study. Am J Surg. 2015;210(6):1118–24; discussion 1124–5.
7. Ewert F, Syed J, Kern S, Besendörfer M, Carbon RT, Schulz-Drost S. Symptoms in pectus deformities: a scoring system for subjective physical complaints. Thorac Cardiovasc Surg. 2017;65(1):43–9.
8. Kelly RE, Cash TF, Shamberger RC, Mitchell KK, Mellins RB, Lawson ML, et al. Surgical repair of pectus excavatum markedly improves body image and perceived ability for physical activity: multicenter study. Pediatrics. 2008;122(6):1218–22.
9. Dupuis, Savina EN, Chavoin J-P, Rivière D, Didier A. Evaluation of quality of life and respiratory function in patients with pectus excavatum. ERS Int Congr; 2017. Milan Themat Poster.
10. Neviere R, Benhamed L, Duva Pentiah A, Wurtz A. Pectus excavatum repair improves respiratory pump efficacy and cardiovascular function at exercise. J Thorac Cardiovasc Surg. 2013;145(2):605–6.
11. Sigalet DL, Montgomery M, Harder J. Cardiopulmonary effects of closed repair of pectus excavatum. J Pediatr Surg. 2003;38(3):380–5; discussion 380–5.
12. Kelly RE, Shamberger RC, Mellins RB, Mitchell KK, Lawson ML, Oldham K, et al. Prospective multicenter study of surgical correction of pectus excavatum: design, perioperative complications, pain, and baseline pulmonary function facilitated by internet-based data collection. J Am Coll Surg. 2007;205(2):205–16.
13. Fonkalsrud EW. 912 open pectus excavatum repairs: changing trends, lessons learned: one surgeon's experience. World J Surg. 2009;33(2):180–90.

14. Kragten HA, Siebenga J, Höppener PF, Verburg R, Visker N. Symptomatic pectus excavatum in seniors (SPES): a cardiovascular problem?: a prospective cardiological study of 42 senior patients with a symptomatic pectus excavatum. Neth Heart J. 2011;19(2):73–8.

15. Kelly RE, Goretsky MJ, Obermeyer R, Kuhn MA, Redlinger R, Haney TS, et al. Twenty-one years of experience with minimally invasive repair of pectus excavatum by the Nuss procedure in 1215 patients. Ann Surg. 2010;252(6):1072–81.

16. Koumbourlis AC, Stolar CJ. Lung growth and function in children and adolescents with idiopathic pectus excavatum. Pediatr Pulmonol. 2004;38(4):339–43.

17. Coskun ZK, Turgut HB, Demirsoy S, Cansu A. The prevalence and effects of pectus excavatum and pectus carinatum on the respiratory function in children between 7-14 years old. Indian J Pediatr. 2010;77(9):1017–9.

18. Lawson ML, Mellins RB, Paulson JF, Shamberger RC, Oldham K, Azizkhan RG, et al. Increasing severity of pectus excavatum is associated with reduced pulmonary function. J Pediatr. 2011;159(2):256–261.e2.

19. Chen Z, Amos EB, Luo H, Su C, Zhong B, Zou J, et al. Comparative pulmonary functional recovery after Nuss and Ravitch procedures for pectus excavatum repair: a meta-analysis. J Cardiothorac Surg. 2012;7:101.

20. Pellegrino R, Viegi G, Brusasco V, Crapo RO, Burgos F, Casaburi R, et al. Interpretative strategies for lung function tests. Eur Respir J. 2005;26(5):948–68.

21. Malek MH, Fonkalsrud EW, Cooper CB. Ventilatory and cardiovascular responses to exercise in patients with pectus excavatum. Chest. 2003;124(3):870–82.

22. Quigley PM, Haller JA, Jelus KL, Loughlin GM, Marcus CL. Cardiorespiratory function before and after corrective surgery in pectus excavatum. J Pediatr. 1996;128(5 Pt 1):638–43.

23. Kowalewski J. Cardiorespiratory function before and after operation for pectus excavatum: medium-term results. Eur J Cardiothorac Surg. 1998;13(3):275–9.

24. Krueger T, Chassot P-G, Christodoulou M, Cheng C, Ris H-B, Magnusson L. Cardiac function assessed by transesophageal echocardiography during pectus excavatum repair. Ann Thorac Surg. 2010;89(1):240–3.

25. Huang P-M, Liu C-M, Cheng Y-J, Kuo S-W, Wu E-T, Lee Y-C. Evaluation of intraoperative cardiovascular responses to closed repair for pectus excavatum. Thorac Cardiovasc Surg. 2008;56(6):353–8.

26. Mocchegiani R, Badano L, Lestuzzi C, Nicolosi GL, Zanuttini D. Relation of right ventricular morphology and function in pectus excavatum to the severity of the chest wall deformity. Am J Cardiol. 1995;76(12):941–6.

27. O'Keefe J, Byrne R, Montgomery M, Harder J, Roberts D, Sigalet DL. Longer term effects of closed repair of pectus excavatum on cardiopulmonary status. J Pediatr Surg. 2013;48(5):1049–54.

28. Tardy MM, Tardy-Médous MM, Filaire M, Patoir A, Gautier-Pignonblanc P, Galvaing G, et al. Exercise cardiac output limitation in pectus excavatum. J Am Coll Cardiol. 2015;66(8):976–7.

29. Borowitz D, Cerny F, Zallen G, Sharp J, Burke M, Gross K, et al. Pulmonary function and exercise response in patients with pectus excavatum after Nuss repair. J Pediatr Surg. 2003;38(4):544–7.

30. Udholm S, Maagaard M, Pilegaard H, Hjortdal V. Cardiac function in adults following minimally invasive repair of pectus excavatum. Interact Cardiovasc Thorac Surg. 2016;22(5):525–9.

31. Castellani C, Schalamon J, Saxena AK, Höellwarth ME. Early complications of the Nuss procedure for pectus excavatum: a prospective study. Pediatr Surg Int. 2008;24(6):659–66.

32. Morshuis WJ, Folgering HT, Barentsz JO, Cox AL, van Lier HJ, Lacquet LK. Exercise cardiorespiratory function before and one year after operation for pectus excavatum. J Thorac Cardiovasc Surg. 1994;107(6):1403–9.

33. Neviere R, Montaigne D, Benhamed L, Catto M, Edme JL, Matran R, et al. Cardiopulmonary response following surgical repair of pectus excavatum in adult patients. Eur J Cardiothorac Surg. 2011;40(2):e77–82.

34. Sigalet DL, Montgomery M, Harder J, Wong V, Kravarusic D, Alassiri A. Long term cardiopulmonary effects of closed repair of pectus excavatum. Pediatr Surg Int. 2007;23(5):493–7.

35. Cahill JL, Lees GM, Robertson HT. A summary of preoperative and postoperative cardiorespiratory performance in patients undergoing pectus excavatum and carinatum repair. J Pediatr Surg. 1984;19(4):430–3.
36. Lomholt JJ, Jacobsen EB, Thastum M, Pilegaard H. A prospective study on quality of life in youths after pectus excavatum correction. Ann Cardiothorac Surg. 2016;5(5):456–65.
37. Kim HK, Shim JH, Choi KS, Choi YH. The quality of life after bar removal in patients after the nuss procedure for pectus excavatum. World J Surg. 2011;35(7):1656–61.
38. Ji Y, Liu W, Chen S, Xu B, Tang Y, Wang X, et al. Assessment of psychosocial functioning and its risk factors in children with pectus excavatum. Health Qual Life Outcomes. 2011;9:28.
39. Chavoin J-P, Grolleau J-L, Moreno B, Brunello J, André A, Dahan M, et al. Correction of pectus excavatum by custom-made silicone implants: contribution of computer-aided design reconstruction. A 20-year experience and 401 cases. Plast Reconstr Surg. 2016;137(5):860e–71e.
40. Steinmann C, Krille S, Mueller A, Weber P, Reingruber B, Martin A. Pectus excavatum and pectus carinatum patients suffer from lower quality of life and impaired body image: a control group comparison of psychological characteristics prior to surgical correction. Eur J Cardiothorac Surg. 2011;40(5):1138–45.
41. Cobben JM, Oostra R-J, van Dijk FS. Pectus excavatum and carinatum. Eur J Med Genet. 2014;57(8):414–7.
42. Vogelmeier CF, Criner GJ, Martínez FJ, Anzueto A, Barnes PJ, Bourbeau J, et al. Global strategy for the diagnosis, management, and prevention of chronic obstructive lung disease 2017 report: GOLD executive summary. Arch Bronconeumol. 2017;53(3):128–49.
43. Global initiative for Asthma. Global strategy for asthma management and prevention; 2017.
44. Kelly RE, Lawson ML, Paidas CN, Hruban RH. Pectus excavatum in a 112-year autopsy series: anatomic findings and the effect on survival. J Pediatr Surg. 2005;40(8):1275–8.

The Cardiorespiratory Implications of Pectus Excavatum

9

Samir S. Shah and Pankaj Kumar Mishra

9.1 Introduction

Pectus excavatum (PE) is a deformity of the sternum, ribs, and the intervening costal cartilages thought to occur as a result of anomalous and asymmetrical costochondral hypertrophy. The pathophysiology of the condition has been extensively studied but the exact aetiology and mechanism giving rise to the defect remains to be definitively established [1].

PE is the most frequently encountered congenital chest wall abnormality with an incidence of between 1 in 300 and 1 in 1000 live births. It predominantly affects males (male/female ratio of 4:1) [2–5]. The condition is known to have a familial component, with nearly half of the patients having a relative with skeletal abnormality, but there is no clear documented genetic link [6, 7].

PE is associated with several heritable connective tissue disorders, such as Marfan's, Ehlers-Danlos, Poland, Mitral valve prolapse, or MASS (Mitral valve prolapse, not progressive Aortic enlargement, Skeletal and Skin alterations) syndromes [8–10]. It is important to note that although PE is frequently encountered in individuals with Marfan's syndrome the converse does not hold true, and in fact, less than 1% patients of PE will have an underlying connective tissue disorder [11]. The association should be acknowledged as some of the connective tissue disorders, Marfan's syndrome, for example, have well-documented cardiopulmonary consequences in their own right.

S. S. Shah (✉) · P. K. Mishra
The Essex Cardiothoracic Centre, Basildon, UK
e-mail: Pankaj.Mishra@btuh.nhs.uk; samir.shah@btuh.nhs.uk

© Springer Nature Switzerland AG 2019
J.-P. Chavoin (ed.), *Pectus Excavatum and Poland Syndrome Surgery*,
https://doi.org/10.1007/978-3-030-05108-2_9

9.2   Cardiopulmonary Implications of PE

The basis of any discussion about the cardiopulmonary implications of PE has to start with the anatomy. The characteristic finding is a depression of the sternum resulting in a decrease in the sterno-vertebral distance in comparison to the transverse diameter of the chest (the basis of the Haller index). This change in the contour of the chest wall, which can be marked, results in the heart being displaced with a variable degree of rotation further into the left hemi-thorax. The right ventricle is the cardiac chamber primarily affected by the altered geometry. The extent is dependent not only on the decrease in the sterno-vertebral distance, but also by the degree of asymmetry present. That is to say, PE is not a deformity affecting the midline. There are other skeletal abnormalities that can co-exist in an individual with PE such as scoliosis of the spine.

The functional significance of the anatomical changes found in PE is an alteration in the cardiopulmonary physiology of the individual. This is brought about in the main by the alteration in the right heart function with a variable degree of impaired diastolic filling. This results in a lower ejection fraction and by definition overall cardiac output secondary to the extrinsic compression.

However, there is uncertainty about the true consequences of these changes and the correlation with the presenting symptomology of patients with PE. In seeking a medical opinion, individuals with PE present with a myriad symptoms. It is often not easy to separate the concerns of the individual with the condition from the "anxieties" of the accompanying parents. The symptoms are however underpinned and dominated by the aesthetic appearance of the chest wall deformity.

Whilst acknowledging the cosmetic significance of PE, the medical fraternity has also attempted to objectively characterize the cardiopulmonary changes associated with PE. The functional significance of the changes has, arguably, formed the basis of justifying the need for surgical intervention beyond simply cosmetic correction.

The most striking thing of note on reviewing the published literature on this subject is the degree of variation, heterogeneity, and the lack of standardization in the great many studies, papers, and reports addressing the cardiopulmonary implications of PE. This is apparent not only in the number of patients included in the studies but also in the demographics of the patient cohorts. There are a number of different surgical techniques employed for the correction of the PE deformity (the description, merits and disadvantages of which are discussed in the relevant chapter). Not surprisingly, these are dependent on the preference of a particular surgeon/surgical group or institution, and yet, the cardiac and pulmonary parameters under investigation have been applied to these different surgical techniques without clear separation. The period of follow-up is also variable from obvious pre- and post-operative changes to only inter-operative changes with little focus on long-term follow-up. Finally, conclusions are reached on the basis of a wide array of investigations from relatively static tests, like simple spirometry and transthoracic or intraoperative transoesophageal echocardiography through to more dynamic and functional assessment of patients using cardiac magnetic resonance imaging

(MRI), cardiopulmonary exercise testing, and optoelectronic plethysmography. This is in part understandable, as there has been great advances in the manner in which we assess both cardiac and pulmonary function and the application of these techniques in different clinical settings.

However, in a recent "best evidence" paper, the extent of heterogeneity in the literature was reflected in the fact that only 22 papers (out of 168 results), of which three were meta-analyses, matched the defined search criteria. An important point of note is that there was no available data from a randomized controlled trial [12–19].

With regard to the pulmonary implications of PE, analysis of the published material suggests that there is a diminution in pulmonary function after surgery for PE particularly in the early post-operative period [20–22]. This may be easy to understand when one considers the technical aspect of the corrective surgery, whether undertaken via a minimally invasive approach (Nuss) or an open correction (Ravitch). The use of "rigid" bars is universal in the Nuss operation and also in the majority of open operations. The presence of a fixed bar is likely to do little to improve the baseline restrictive nature of chest wall movement associated with PE. A study of seven patients, in whom optoelectronic plethysmography was utilized, demonstrated reduced ribcage mobility after Nuss correction [20]. This explanation is further supported by improvement in lung function on removal of the bar [12, 19, 23]. However, by the same token, there are many studies which have either reported no long-term improvement in pulmonary function or that any improvement never exceeds the preoperative baseline [17, 24, 25].

In contrast to this mixed picture, there would appear to be a clear, definite, and sustained improvement in the cardiac function of individuals who have undergone surgical correction of a PE deformity. Moreover, as the detail and intricacy of the assessment of cardiac function has improved, particularly in the form of detailed echocardiography and cardiac MRI, this finding is consistent across a number of different imaging modalities [26, 27].

Transoesophageal echocardiography speckle-tracking strain and strain rate, used to evaluate and detect subclinical myocardial dysfunction in patients receiving cardiotoxic chemotherapy and those with valvular heart disease, was applied to investigate the effects of PE surgery on right (RV) and left (LV) ventricular function. The study demonstrated significant improvement in both RV and LV longitudinal strain and strain rate following PE repair using a modified or hybrid Nuss procedure [28, 29]. Furthermore, there was a strong correlation between the degree of right atrial compression and the RV strain [26].

These findings are supported by the changes observed in pre- and post-operative RV and LV ejection fraction on cardiac MRI. Both were reduced prior to surgery but not only improved immediately after surgery but this improvement was sustained at 1-year follow-up. Interestingly, although the increase in ejection fraction was small it was significant only as far as RV function was concerned whereas that of the LV did not attain statistical significance [27].

Other studies have reported that the surgical correction of PE improves diastolic filling of the heart, specifically the RV, and results in an increase in RV cardiac output of 38%; this increase is more marked (65% increase) in older patients (those greater than 30 years of age) [30, 31]. Furthermore, the increase in stroke volume/ejection fraction is observed both in patients subject to the minimally invasive Nuss procedure and the open Ravitch operation [13, 21, 32].

The purported mechanism by which this is achieved is thought secondary to the alleviation of the external compression of the RV that occurs directly as a result of the PE deformity.

In the cardiac surgery setting, the presence of right ventricular dysfunction or failure either preoperatively (e.g. secondary to pulmonary hypertension) or post-operatively in instances where there may have been a problem with intra-operative myocardial protection, can result in difficult post-operative course in patients and can be a negative prognostic factor on outcome following a cardiac operation. Indeed, arguably in some cases, evidence of severe right ventricular dysfunction may preclude cardiac surgical intervention altogether in the same manner as poor left ventricular ejection fraction does at times.

However, quite what the finding of right ventricular impairment heralds prognostically in the context of an individual with a PE deformity remains to be clarified. The compression is extrinsic and the repair of the PE deformity does not interfere with the heart (unless it is injured during minimally invasive surgery for PE). On a point of caution, if a patient is undergoing a cardiac surgical operation with a concomitant and significant PE deformity, it may be prudent to consider repairing the latter to prevent any problems secondary to the "mechanical" compression of the right ventricle.

Most of the reported literature related to the cardiopulmonary impact of PE pertains to adolescents and young adults. In this group of individuals, the leftward deviation of the heart coupled with a compliant thoracic cage can confer some protection from the overt effects of cardiac compression. In this group of individuals, symptoms suggestive of cardiorespiratory dysfunction, such as dyspnoea on exertion, are often only apparent at a high level of exertion. However, this situation changes considerably in individuals in later life when the chest becomes stiff and non-compliant. There have been reports of cardiac failure in older patients (beyond the fifth decade of life) secondary to symptomatic PE (and in whom other causes of cardiac failure like ischaemic heart disease have been excluded). These patients have attained significant symptomatic, functional, and clinical relief following the surgical correction of PE deformity [33–35].

The overwhelming emphasis in the literature is focused on cardiopulmonary effects of PE. There is a particular bias on the manner in which corrective surgery for the condition potentially improves the cardiopulmonary function. It is important to consider the physiological implications of not operating on individuals with PE. One such study reported a 10-year follow-up of 75 patients with PE, of whom 37 patients underwent surgical repair and 38 patients who did not have an operation [36]. The results demonstrated that in "non-operated" individuals there was an improvement in both sterno-vertebral measurement (in centimetres) and respiratory function (the operated group experienced a deterioration in lung function consistent with studies alluded to earlier). Furthermore, there was no difference in the measured functional and work performance parameters after 10 years between the two groups. It is possible that not all individuals with PE require corrective surgery, and this is important to bear in mind in the management of the condition.

9.3   Conclusion

There is more to PE than meets the eye though equally, it is the visual consequence that troubles those afflicted with the condition. Few would argue that in the majority of instances it is the aesthetic appearance that is not only a major impediment to the psychological well-being and the physical prowess of the individual with PE, but also the driving force in seeking medical assistance. There is no doubt that the surgical correction of the condition, including techniques involving bespoke silicone implants, produces good results and caters admirably for the cosmetic and well-being aspect of individuals [37].

The more complex area of debate and discussion relates to whether PE can be described as a pathological condition in the same vein as other conditions that have the potential to have detrimental health consequences if left uncorrected.

There is a great deal of information about the physiological impact of PE, and it is exclusively focused on the cardiopulmonary sequelae of the condition. The body of information is being added to at an inexorable pace but the true relevance of the findings remains to be clearly delineated. It is important that the clinicians driving the research retain objectivity when it comes to assessing the available information. This would help to define more clearly patients in whom surgery is undertaken for purely cosmetic reasons from those who merit an operation for clinical reasons. Surgery on the basis of the Haller index is arguably no longer valid.

Healthcare economies around the world are under increasing pressure to commission only evidence-based treatments. On reviewing the literature, there is a perception that studies are being performed as a means to justify an end and the fact that many reports are inadequately powered together with the absence of true long-term follow-up, and perhaps, most telling of all the absence of a randomized controlled trial simply adds to this perception.

References

1. Tocchioni F, Ghionzoli M, Messineo A, et al. Pectus excavatum and heritable disorders of the connective tissue. Pediatr Rep. 2013;5(3):e15.
2. Williams AM, Crabbe DC. Pectus deformities of the anterior chest wall. Paediatr Respir Rev. 2003;4:237–42.
3. Tocchioni F, Ghionzoli M, Pepe G, et al. Pectus excavatum and MASS phenotype: an unknown association. J Laparoendosc Adv Surg Tech A. 2012;22:508–13.
4. Cartoski MJ, Nuss D, Goretsky MJ, et al. Classification of the dysmorphology of pectus excavatum. J Pediatr Surg. 2006;41:1573–81.
5. Rattan AS, Laor T, Ryckman FC, et al. Pectus excavatum imaging: enough but not too much. Pediatr Radiol. 2012;40:168–72.
6. Creswick HA, Stacey MW, Kelly RE Jr, et al. Family study of the inheritance of pectus excavatum. J Pediatr Surg. 2006;41:1699–703.

7. Jaroszewski D, Notrica D, McMahon L, et al. Current management of pectus excavatum: a review and update of therapy and treatment recommendations. J Am Board Fam Med. 2010;23:230–9.
8. Redlinger RE Jr, Rushing GD, Moskowitz AD, et al. Minimally invasive repair of pectus excavatum in patients with Marfan syndrome and marfanoid features. J Pediatr Surg. 2010;45:193–9.
9. Ho NC, Tran JR, Bektas A. Marfan's syndrome. Lancet. 2005;366:1978–81.
10. Le Parc JM, Molcard S, Tubach F, et al. Marfan syndrome and fibrillin disorders. Joint Bone Spine. 2000;67:401–7.
11. Colombani PM. Preoperative assessment of chest wall deformities. Semin Thorac Cardiovasc Surg. 2009;21:58–63.
12. Jayaramakrishnan K, Wotton R, Bradley A, et al. Does repair of pectus excavatum improve cardiopulmonary function? Interact Cardiovasc Thorac Surg. 2013;16(6):865–70.
13. Malek MH, Berger DE, Marelich WD, et al. Pulmonary function following surgical repair of pectus excavatum: a meta-analysis. Eur J Cardiothorac Surg. 2006;30:637–43.
14. Malek MH, Berger DE, Housh TJ, et al. Cardiovascular function following surgical repair of pectus excavatum: a meta-analysis. Chest. 2006;130:506–16.
15. Johnson JN, Hartman TK, Pianosi PT, et al. Cardiorespiratory function after operation for pectus excavatum. J Pediatr. 2008;153:359–64.
16. Coln E, Carrasco J, Coln D. Demonstrating relief of cardiac compression with the Nuss minimally invasive repair for pectus excavatum. J Pediatr Surg. 2006;41:683–6.
17. Castellani C, Windhaber J, Schober PH, et al. Exercise performance testing in patients with pectus excavatum before and after Nuss procedure. Pediatr Surg Int. 2010;26:659–63.
18. Tang M, Nielson HH, Lesbo M, et al. Improved cardiopulmonary exercise function after modified Nuss operation for pectus excavatum. Eur J Cardiothorac Surg. 2012;41:1063–7.
19. Sigalet DL, Montgomery M, Harder J, et al. Long term cardiopulmonary effects of closed repair of pectus excavatum. Pediatr Surg Int. 2007;23:493–7.
20. Acosta J, Bradley A, Raja V, et al. Exercise improvement after pectus excavatum repair is not related to chest wall function. Eur J Cardiothorac Surg. 2014;45(3):544–8.
21. Sigalet DL, Montgomery M, Harder J. Cardiopulmonary effects of closed repair of pectus excavatum. J Pediatr Surg. 2003;38:380–5.
22. Borowitz D, Cerny F, Zallen G, et al. Pulmonary function and exercise response in patients with pectus excavatum after Nuss repair. J Pediatr Surg. 2003;38:544–7.
23. Lawson ML, Mellins RB, Tabangin M, et al. Impact of pectus excavatum on pulmonary function before and after repair with the Nuss procedure. J Pediatr Surg. 2005;40:174–80.
24. Bawazir OA, Montgomery M, Harder J, et al. Midterm evaluation of cardiopulmonary effects of closed repair for pectus excavatum. J Pediatr Surg. 2005;40:863–7.
25. Udholm S, Maagaard M, Pilegaard H, et al. Cardiac function in adults following minimally invasive repair of pectus excavatum. Interact Cardiovasc Thorac Surg. 2016;22(5):525–9.
26. Chao CJ, Dawn Jaroszewski D, Gotway M, et al. Effects of pectus excavatum repair on right and left ventricular strain. Ann Thorac Surg. 2018;105:294–301.
27. Topper A, Polleichtner S, Zagrosek A, et al. Impact of surgical correction of pectus excavatum on cardiac function: insights on the right ventricle. A cardiovascular magnetic resonance study. Interact Cardiovasc Thorac Surg. 2016;22:38–46.
28. Nuss D. Minimally invasive surgical repair of pectus excavatum. Semin Pediatr Surg. 2008;17:209–17.
29. Jaroszewski DE, Fonkalsrud EW. Repair of pectus chest wall deformities in 320 adult patients: 21-year experience. Ann Thorac Surg. 2007;84:429–33.
30. Jaroszewski DE. Physiologic implications of pectus excavatum. J Thorac Cardiovasc Surg. 2017;153:218–9.
31. Chao CJ, Jaroszewski DE, Kumar PN, et al. Surgical repair of pectus excavatum relieves right heart chamber compression and improves cardiac output in adult patients—an intraoperative transesophageal echocardiographic study. Am J Surg. 2015;210:1118–24; discussion 1124–5.

32. Quigley PM, Haller JA Jr, Jelus KL, et al. Cardiorespiratory function before and after corrective surgery in pectus excavatum. J Pediatr. 1996;128:638–43.
33. Winkens R, Guldemond F, Hoppener P, et al. Pectus excavatum, not always as harmless as it seems. BMJ Case Rep. 2009.
34. Jaroszewski D, Steidley E, Galindo A, et al. Treating heart failure and dyspnoea in a 78-year-old man with surgical correction of pectus excavatum. Ann Thorac Surg. 2009;88:1008–10.
35. Kragten HA, Siebenga J, Höppener PF, et al. Symptomatic pectus excavatum in seniors (SPES): a cardiovascular problem? A prospective cardiological study of 42 senior patients with a symptomatic pectus excavatum. Neth Heart J. 2011;19:73–8.
36. Gyllensward A, Irnell L, Michaelsson M, et al. Pectus excavatum. A clinical study with long term postoperative follow-up. Acta Paediatr Scand. 1975;255(Suppl):1–14.
37. Chavoin JP, Grolleau JL, Moreno B, et al. Correction of pectus excavatum by custom-made silicone implants: contribution of computer-aided design reconstruction. A 20-year experience and 401 cases. Plast Reconstr Surg. 2016;137:860e–71e.

Complications and Hazards with Pectus Excavatum Surgeries: Secondary Surgical Procedures with Implants

10

Françoise Le Pimpec Barthes, Ian Hunt, Samir S. Shah, Antonio Messineo, Louis Daussy, Aymeric André, Marcel Dahan, and Jean-Pierre Chavoin

F. Le Pimpec Barthes (✉)
Thoracic and Pulmonary Surgery Department, Georges-Pompidou European Hospital AP-HP, Paris, France
e-mail: francoise.lepimpec-barthes@aphp.fr

I. Hunt
Pectus Clinic, London, UK
e-mail: enquires@pectusclinic.com

S. S. Shah
The Essex Cardiothoracic Centre, Basildon, UK
e-mail: samir.shah@btuh.nhs.uk

A. Messineo
Pediatric Surgery Department, AOU Meyer, Florence, Italy
e-mail: antonio.messineo@meyer.it

L. Daussy
Pulmonary Department, Albi Hospital, Albi, France
e-mail: louis.daussy@outlook.fr

A. André
Plastic Surgery Department, Rangueil Hospital, Toulouse University Hospital, Toulouse, France

M. Dahan
Thoracic Surgery Department, Larrey Hospital, Toulouse University Hospital, Toulouse, France
e-mail: dahan.m@chu-toulouse.fr

J.-P. Chavoin
Plastic Surgery Department, Rangueil Hospital, Toulouse University Hospital, Toulouse, France
e-mail: jean-pierre.chavoin@orange.fr

© Springer Nature Switzerland AG 2019
J.-P. Chavoin (ed.), *Pectus Excavatum and Poland Syndrome Surgery*,
https://doi.org/10.1007/978-3-030-05108-2_10

10.1 Introduction

The analysis of the literature and the experience of thoracic, paediatric, and plastic surgeons show that there are some questions regarding procedures such as direct orthopaedic remodelling of the thorax, either through open techniques or so called mini invasive technic endoscopically controlled.

The problem is for patients whose main wish is to have a normal chest profile without pain and risks, but also for the surgeon who never likes stress and heavy complications, and even poor results.

10.2 Morbidity and Mortality of Procedures Correcting the Deformation

10.2.1 Common Complications to Both Corrective Surgeries

A meta-analysis published in 2016 by Kanagaratnam et al. [1] reports and compares the rate of occurrence of the most frequently encountered complications. It includes the results of 13 studies comprising a total of 1432 patients in paediatric, mixed, and adult populations. However, there is a majority of minor patients (80%) compared to adults (only 20%).

The overall rate of complications in all populations (paediatric, mixed, and adult) was 14% for Ravitch procedure and 28.2% for Nuss procedure although no statistically significant difference was found (OR = 1.58, 95% CI: 0.86–2.90, I2 = 62%, $P = 0.14$). The rate of early complications would be lower with Ravitch procedure in mixed and adult cohorts.

Movement of osteosynthesis material was significantly lower in patients who underwent Ravitch procedure (OR = 4.17, 95% CI: 1.46–11.96, I2 = 0%, $P = 0.008$) (Figs. 10.1, 10.2, and 10.3).

The rate of surgical revision in all populations combined was 3.3% for Ravitch procedure and 7.7% for Nuss procedure without a statistically significant difference being found. One exception was the subgroup of adult patients in which the rate was significantly lower in the Ravitch group compared to the Nuss group (5.4% vs. 28.6%, OR = 7.07, 95% CI: 1.37–36.52, $P = 0.02$).

The rate of surgical site infections was 1.7% for Ravitch procedure and 1.3% for Nuss procedure.

The haemothorax rate in all populations was 0.8% in the Ravitch group and 1.3% in the Nuss group.

The rate of pneumothorax in all populations combined was 2.1% in the Ravitch group and 4.2% in the Nuss group.

No significant difference was found between the two surgeries with respect to the rate of surgical site infections, haemothorax.

There was no statistically significant difference between the two techniques with respect to pneumonia, which was otherwise very low (Nuss, 0.1%; Ravitch, 0.7%).

Fig. 10.1 Ravitch's bar displacement on the right lung

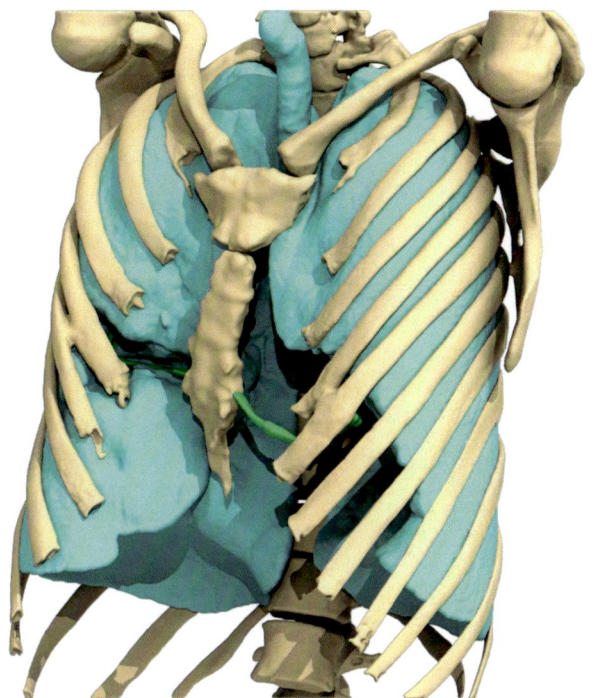

Fig. 10.2 Nuss's bar displacement into the right lung without correction

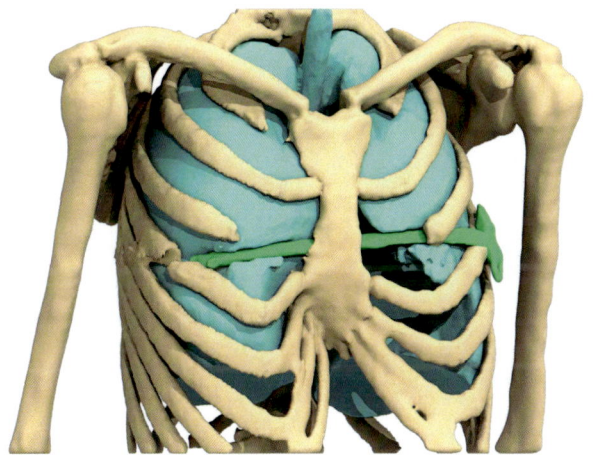

The recurrence rate of PE is a complication described in both Nuss and Ravitch procedures. In the retrospective study of Tikka et al. (2016) (169 PE, 116 FP, mean follow-up 8.6 years), the rate reached 10% [2]. For patients with PE, the rate was 2% ($n = 1/50$) for Nuss procedure and 18% for Ravitch procedure with stabilizer splint ($n = 12/66$) and 8% ($n = 4/50$) without splint. Univariate analysis also showed that patients developing postoperative complications were more likely to have recurrence (Figs. 10.4 and 10.5).

Fig. 10.3 Double
fractured Ravitch's bar

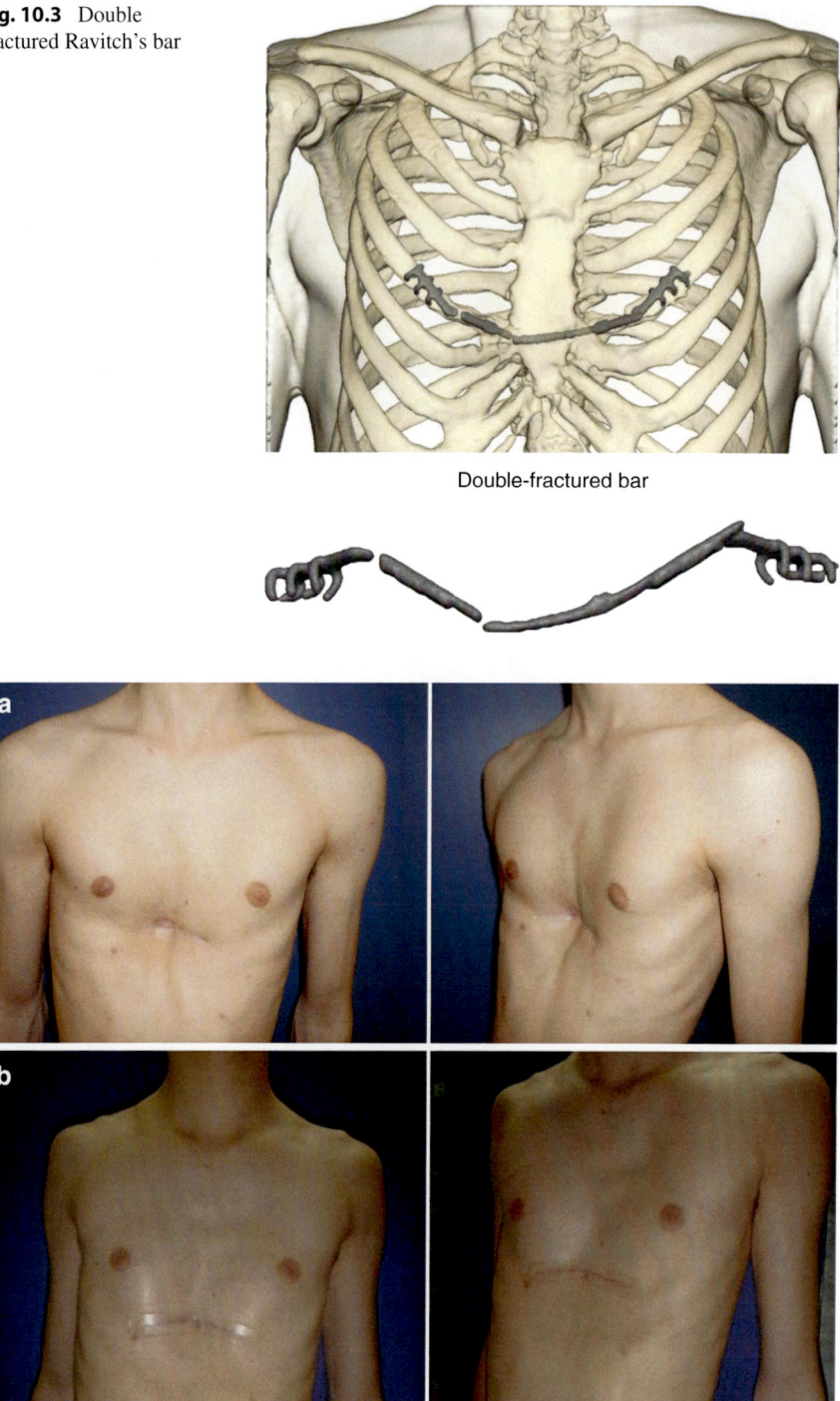

Double-fractured bar

Fig. 10.4 (**a**) Ravitch's partial recurrence. (**b**) Early result after CAD implant procedure (**c**) Implant's digital image front face. (**d**) Implant's digital image in supine position

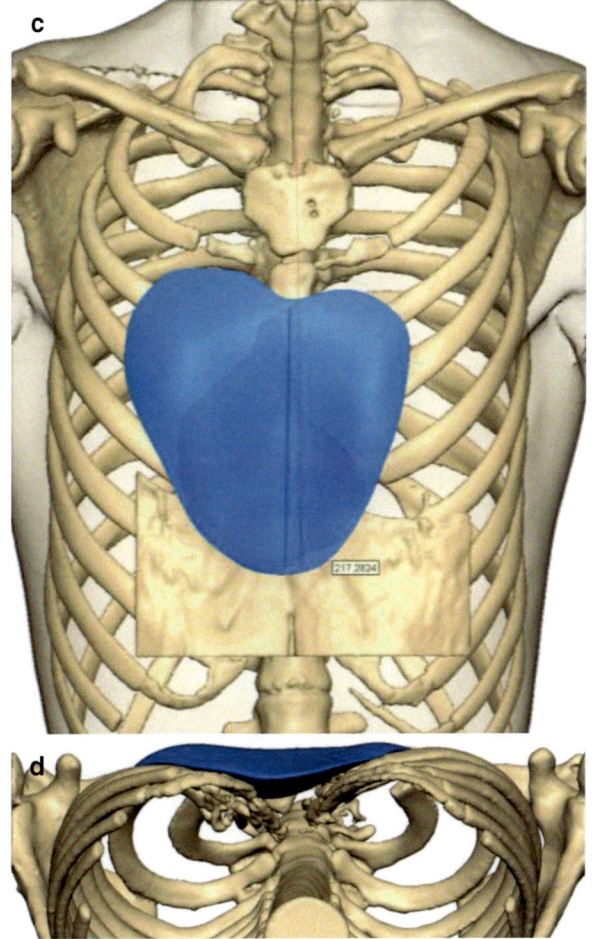

Fig. 10.4 (continued)

10.2.2 Complications Specific to Ravitch Procedure

10.2.2.1   Scar Dystrophy

The scar from Ravitch procedure is long and sometimes dehiscent (Fig. 10.6).

10.2.2.2   Restricted Thoracic Dystrophy

Some patients operated on during childhood developed a severe deficit in the growth of the ribcage responsible for the restrictive ventilatory defects, which sometimes is severe. This phenomenon was found by Haller in 1995 [3] who described in several young patients a severe deterioration of their ventilatory capacity ranging from 30 to 50% and their FEV1 from 25 to 55% in patients with severe disabilities. He explained this phenomenon by relating to the fact that these patients had been

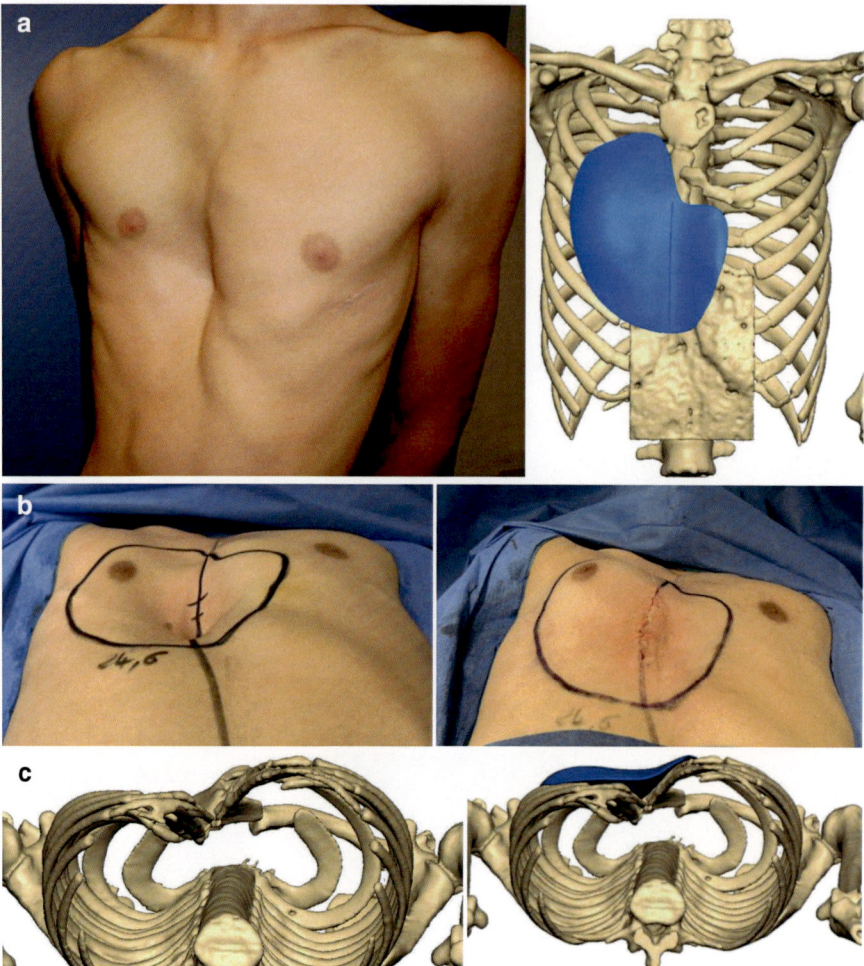

Fig. 10.5 (**a**) Recurrence after Nuss preop, CAD project front face. (**b**) Implant's correction preop. (**c**) CAD project in supine position

operated too young (2–6 years old) and had undergone too extensive cartilaginous resection (5 or more). There is no doubt that the "bridges" procedure with four bars prevents any movement of the bars but yields breathing growing and playing problematic for young patients currently operated before 10 (11).

In 2004, Robicsek et al. [4] warned again about this phenomenon, which they call ARTD ("acquired restrictive thoracic dystrophy"), and they consider not operating patients who are too young and pointed on the faults in the surgical technique. These faults were chondro-costal extractions with removal of the ossification centres and poor suture of the perichondrium retrosternal, responsible for the growth of cartilage behind the sternum. Thanks to the development of surgical technique, to the experience of surgeons, and to the setting of a minimum age of 12 years for surgical operation, this complication has no longer been described in the literature.

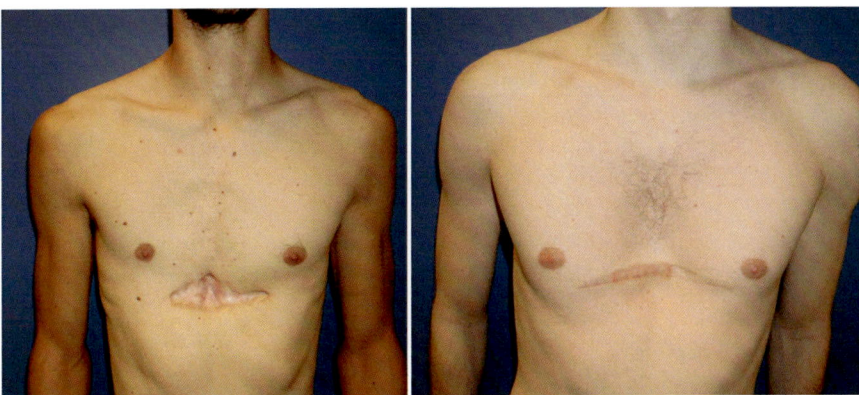

Fig. 10.6 Dehiscent scars after Ravitch procedure

However, this phenomenon seems to be still present although to a much lesser extent and without significant consequences. This is illustrated by the study of Morshuis et al. [5] in adolescents (15 patients, 6 controls, 15 ± 3 years) who found at 1 year of surgery that FVC decreased from 81 ± 17% to 80 ± 16% in the PE group, while it increased in the control group (93 ± 8% ≥ 97 ± 7%). Nevertheless, this difference was not statistically significant. Neviere et al. [6] also found this phenomenon in 70 adult patients (27 ± 11 years) with a statistically significant decrease in FVC of 2 ± 7% (P 0.058), FEV1 of 3 ± 6% (P: 0.006), or CPT of 2 ± 7% (P 0.013%).

10.2.2.3 Wound Haemorrhage of the Phrenic Artery [7]

A 15 years old patient operated 3 months earlier by Ravitch procedure with splinting equipment was diagnosed with haemothorax. The mechanism was laceration of the artery by migration of the material. The evolution was favourable after surgical revision consisting of ligating the artery and removing the material.

10.2.3 Complications Specific to Nuss Procedure

10.2.3.1 Cardiovascular Complications

Difficulties in Practising a Classic Cardiopulmonary Resuscitation [8]

In 2005 Garret et al. published a clinical case of cardiac arrest in a 19-year-old man at 35 months after Nuss procedure. Unfortunately, resuscitation, which included cardiac massage and external electrical shocks due to the diagnosis of ventricular fibrillation, failed to recover the patient. The autopsy did not show any argument for possible cardiac damage related to the position of the bar and it was concluded as ventricular arrhythmia on cardiopathy. Arrhythmia on the stress test, premature ventricular complexes on the ECG, a prolapse of the mitral valve and mild aortic insufficiency had been identified in this patient during preoperative assessment and an ECG Holter was programmed. Note that the patient had not been diagnosed previously with Marfan syndrome.

If the probability of recovering a cardiac arrest is low, about 3%, the authors warn that the Nuss bar could compromise the resuscitation in two ways; firstly, by limiting the essential thoracic depression for an effective cardiac massage, difficulty indicated by the "paramedics" who started resuscitation, and secondly, by the fact the external electric shock had no path possibly to cross the heart because it would have been driven mainly by the metal bar.

In 2003, a communication from the journal *Resuscitation* suggested that some peculiarities of management concerning the cardiopulmonary resuscitation of patients operated by Nuss technique with notably: placement of defibrillator pallets in anteroposterior and not in anterolateral position and early exclusion of the diagnosis of pneumothorax that could be related to the displacement of the bar [9].

Heart Perforations

The risk of cardiac injury can occur during the operation of the retrosternal space dissection, the introduction of the bar, and its progression in this region. It can also occur remotely from surgery due to the migration of the bar. The systematic use of a thoracoscopic check did not make it possible to eliminate this type of intraoperative complication, the consequences of which are often very serious.

The clinical case reported by Schaarschmidt et al. [10] in 2013 illustrates this well. It was a Nuss procedure performed in 2006 by a trained team under double thoracoscopic control. While the surgeons had not encountered any particular difficulties during surgery, except for a pericardium that seemed a little more adherent to the sternum than usual and that the procedure was almost complete, the patient had a cardiac arrest. The surgery quickly converted to open chest surgery, identifying two wounds of about 7 mm from the right atrium and right ventricle that were sutured. The patient finally died on day 11 of major cerebral oedema complicated by the low flow rate caused by the 30 min perioperative cardiopulmonary resuscitation necessary to stabilize his haemodynamic state.

Their review of the literature listed the described cases of post-traumatic cardiac complications of Nuss procedure, intraoperative [10–13] and early postoperative, and late removal of the bar or during migration. The review also included 13 cases of cardiac lesions in patients aged 8–18 years who reported three lethal cases as well as cases of severe brain complications after cardiac resuscitation is performed.

Haemorrhagic Shock on Arterial Lesions

A case of haemorrhagic shock with tamponade in a 17-year-old patient after 2 months of surgery which required an early operative restart for bar displacement was described. The haemorrhagic shock was related to a 1.5 cm wound of the ascending aorta caused by a new migration of the bar requiring removal and a suture of the aorta [12].

Cases of haemorrhagic shock in connection with a wound on the right internal mammary artery in patients aged 13–19 years have also been described. In one case, the table was intraoperative and required ligation of the artery and transfusion [14]. In two other cases, it occurred several months after the surgery (M3 and M4) and required a diagnostic thoracoscopy and an arterio-embolization treatment for the first one [15] and a thoracotomy for local treatment of the injured artery and a with-drawal of the bar for the second [16].

Mechanical Occlusion of the Inferior Vena Cava
This is a very rare complication that has only been described twice in the literature. It occurred in a 13-year-old patient who presented a hypovolaemic shock immediately following Nuss procedure, caused by direct compression of the liver by the bar, which itself compressed the inferior vena cava in its intrahepatic portion [17]. The second, published in 2012, concerned a 15-year-old man [18]. In both cases, the evolution was favourable after surgical recovery for removal of the bar.

Reactive Pericarditis [19]
The mechanism seems to be more often a contact allergy to a bar metal, especially nickel, than an irritative contact phenomenon. In the cohort of 1215 patients operated by Kelly et al. between 1987 and 2008, pericarditis occurred in five patients (0.5%). Three of them required the removal of the metal bar whose two cases with rest of a titanium bar and one without.

10.2.3.2   Pleural Complications
Pneumothorax is a frequent and almost inevitable complication of the technique. The introduction of a positive expiratory pressure (PEP) at the end of the procedure makes it possible to reapply the pleura to the chest wall and thus prevent the formation of a pneumothorax or limit its extent. It is particularly common postoperatively (present in nearly 65% of cases), but is usually of low incidence, clinically well tolerated, and spontaneously resolving. However, it requires drainage management in 4% of cases [19].

Pleural effusions requiring drainage occur in 0.3–0.9% of cases [19, 20].

Haemothorax is most often secondary to an arterial lesion, for example, the internal mammary artery as previously described. It can occur in the early postoperative period (<1 month) or as a late complication with an identified leading cause (trauma) or not. The haemothorax rate is 1.3% in the meta-analysis of Kanagaratnam et al. [1]. In Kelly's study, it occurred early in 0.5% of cases and late in 0.4% of cases [21].

10.2.3.3   Allergic Complications
This rare complication can be manifested only in erythema and local rash. It is sometimes associated with cough or chest pain, in connection with pleural and/or pericardial effusions consecutive to a contact allergy.

In Kelly et al. [19], nickel contact allergy was found in 35 patients (2.8%), of whom 22 were identified to have received a titanium bar. Of the remaining 13 patients, 10 were successfully treated with prednisone and 3 required removal of the bar.

10.2.3.4   Complications Related to Instability, Fracture, or Displacement of Osteosynthesis Material
Displacement of the bar is a relatively common complication of this surgery. If in most of the cases it causes only a defect or a lack of results, it can lead to more

serious complications such as intra-costal migrations [22], trans-sternal thymec-tomy [23], lesion of the left ventricle [24], internal mammary artery injury [16], and aortic injury [25]. Kelly et al. [19] reported a 5.7% displacement rate, of which 4% required surgical revision. The optimization of the costal fixation technique of the bar has reduced its incidence, from 12% in the first decade to 2% over the last 5 years (Figs. 10.1 and 10.2).

10.2.3.5 Nervous Complications

Thoraco-brachial parade syndrome is a common complication affecting 15% of men and one third of women in the Nagasao et al. retrospective study published in 2017 [26].

Transient paralysis of the upper limbs has been described, occurring postopera-tively in the setting or after removal of the Nuss bar [12]. They were related to intra-operative plexus-brachial compression by the head of the humerus due to a poor patient position. A modification of the installation technique proposed by Fox et al. [27] in an article published in 2005 would reduce this complication from 5.8 to 0%.

10.2.3.6 Osteoarticular Complications

A sternal fracture complicating a migration of the bar across the sternum has been described in a 21-year-old woman with a history of Marfan syndrome and Ravitch procedure at age 10 [23].

Peterson et al. [28] described a case of bilateral sternal disjunction during a Nuss surgical revision motivated by bar mobilization in a 13-year-old patient.

10.2.3.7 Infectious Complications

The rate of infectious complications following Nuss procedure is between 1 and 6.8% in the literature. In their article specifically dedicated to this complication with a rate of 1.5%, Shin et al. [29] described 6 bar infections, 4 parietal cellulitis, and 3 cutaneous abscesses on the sutures. Bar infections were defined by the presence of an abscess in contact with the bar. While surgical drainage combined with pro-longed antibiotic therapy effectively treated these three infections, the remaining three required early removal of equipment.

10.2.3.8 Pain

The early postoperative pain of Nuss procedure is particularly intense [30]. Prolonged postoperative chest pain is also observed in the clinical setting in a sig-nificant proportion of patients, but there is very little data available in the literature. In the Kelly et al. multicentre study, which consisted mainly of patients who had undergone Nuss procedure, 1.5% had pain that persisted for more than 1 month after surgery. The mechanism of this prolonged pain, which sometimes requires removal of the bar, seems to be related to the mechanical stress applied to the sterno-chondro-costal chest by the bar, the force of which can reach up to 200 N in children and up to 250 N in adults [31]. This would explain why pain is greater, extended, and prolonged in adults than in children [26].

10.2.3.9   Over-correction of the Deformation

It corresponds to an excessive correction of the deformation at the origin of the transformation of PE into pectus carinatum and therefore of a bad aesthetic result. Its rate was 3.5% in the 2010 Kelly et al. publication [19] (Fig. 10.7).

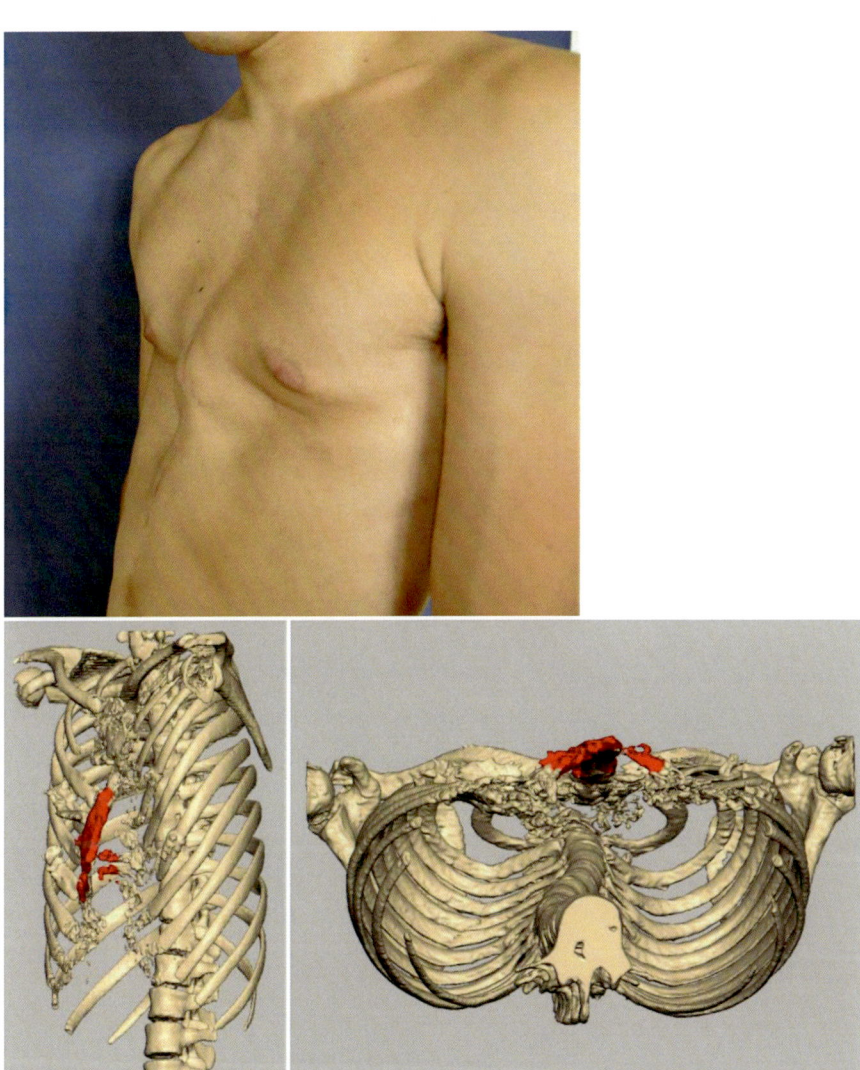

Fig. 10.7 Over-correction after a Ravitch's procedure: CAD project to cut the excess of protuding sternum (*in red*), (allowing to put a custom-made implant on the new thorax surface to correct the remaining pectus excavatum)

10.3   Morbidity and Mortality of Prof. Chavoin's CAD Custom-Made Implant Procedure

The complications are mentioned in the article published by Chavoin et al. [32] concerning nearly 401 patients who benefited from the technique and had custom-made plaster mould implant ($n = 61/15\%$) or custom-made CT scan implant ($n = 340/85\%$) over an average follow-up period of 98 months and 45 months, respectively.

The most common complication was subcutaneous seroma, which affected all patients and was resolute after typically 2–3 punctures.

Other complications identified were:

- Three haematomas (0.75%), related to a lesion of the perforating internal mammary artery, during the intraoperative dissection of the pectoralis major muscle, requiring reoperation
- A late prosthetic infection (0.2%), 7 years after management, requiring its removal
- Two cases (0.5%) of postoperative dehiscence of the scar effectively treated with a new suture

This procedure is used more and more to correct the poor results or failure of other invasive techniques (Figs. 10.8 and 10.9).

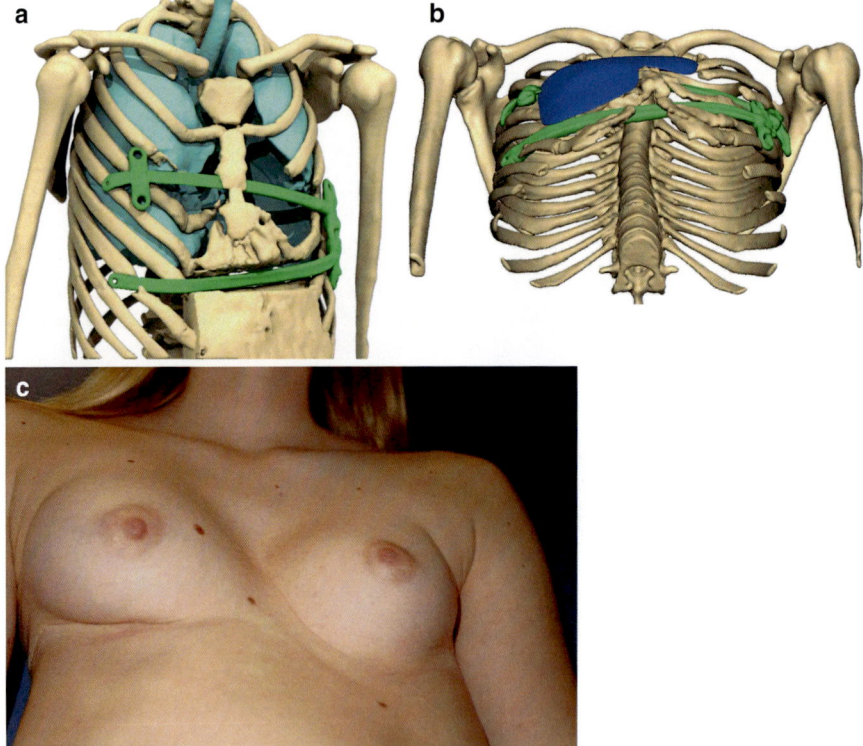

Fig. 10.8 Nuss procedures two poor results to be corrected by a custom made implant: (**a–b**) two bars and CAD implant project. (**c**) Another clinical case with remaining breast asymmetry to be corrected with implant

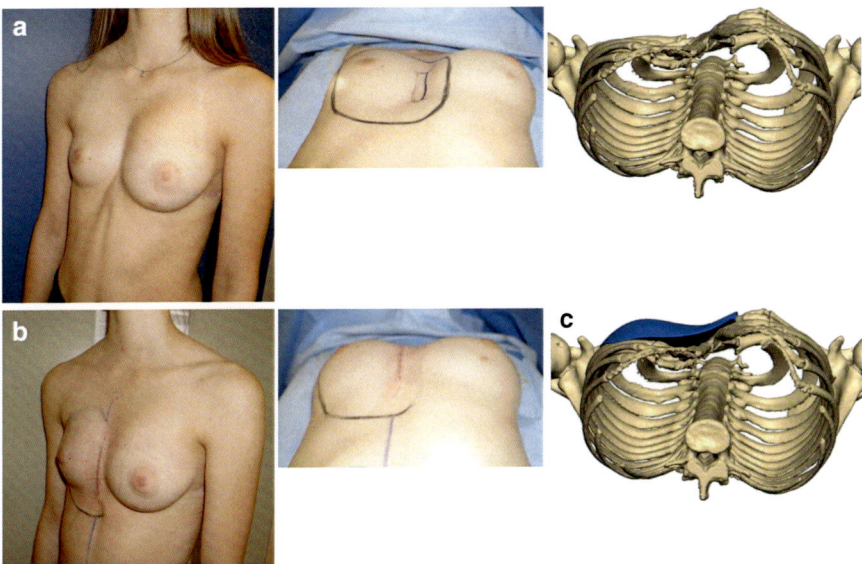

Fig. 10.9 Secondary procedure with CAD implant after Nuss bar migration. (**a**) Preoperative view. (**b**) Postoperative view. (**c**) CAD in supine position

10.4 Conclusion

The complication rate varies a lot from one technique to another with much more frequent complications for corrective surgeries, in particular for Nuss procedure, with significant consequences (complementary invasive care, operative revision, life-threatening procedure). This raises the question of the benefit/risk ratio of such surgeries compared to the CAD silicone custom-made implant technique when the demand is solely or mainly aesthetic.

References

1. Kanagaratnam A, Phan S, Tchantchaleishvili V, Phan K. Ravitch versus Nuss procedure for pectus excavatum: systematic review and meta-analysis. Ann Cardiothorac Surg. 2016;5(5):409–21.
2. Tikka T, Kalkat MS, Bishay E, Steyn RS, Rajesh PB, Naidu B. A 20-year review of pectus surgery: an analysis of factors predictive of recurrence and outcomes. Interact Cardiovasc Thorac Surg. 2016;23(6):908–13.
3. Haller J. Severe chest wall construction from growth retardation after too extensive and too early (<4 years) pectus excavatum repair: an alert. Ann Thorac Surg. 1995;60:1857–8.
4. Robicsek F, Fokin AA. How not to do it: restrictive thoracic dystrophy after pectus excavatum repair. Interact Cardiovasc Thorac Surg. 2004;3(4):566–8.
5. Morshuis WJ, Folgering HT, Barentsz JO, Cox AL, van Lier HJ, Lacquet LK. Exercise cardiorespiratory function before and one year after operation for pectus excavatum. J Thorac Cardiovasc Surg. 1994;107(6):1403–9.

6. Neviere R, et al. Cardiopulmonary response following surgical repair of pectus excavatum in adult patients. Eur J Cardiothorac Surg. 2011;40(2):e77–82.
7. Paret G, Taustein I, Vardi A, Yellin A, Dekel B, Barzilay Z. Laceration of the phrenic artery. A life-threatening complication after repair of pectus excavatum. J Cardiovasc Surg (Torino). 1996;37(2):193–4.
8. Zoeller GK, Zallen GS, Glick PL. Cardiopulmonary resuscitation in patients with a Nuss bar—a case report and review of the literature. J Pediatr Surg. 2005;40(11):1788–91.
9. Picton P, Walker D, White N, Deakin C. Cardiopulmonary resuscitation following minimally invasive repair of pectus excavatum (Nuss technique). Resuscitation. 2003;57(3):309–10.
10. Schaarschmidt K, Lempe M, Schlesinger F, Jaeschke U, Park W, Polleichtner S. Lessons learned from lethal cardiac injury by Nuss repair of pectus excavatum in a 16-year-old. Ann Thorac Surg. 2013;95(5):1793–5.
11. Park HJ, Lee SY, Lee CS. Complications associated with the Nuss procedure: analysis of risk factors and suggested measures for prevention of complications. J Pediatr Surg. 2004;39(3):391–5.
12. Castellani C, Schalamon J, Saxena AK, Höellwarth ME. Early complications of the Nuss procedure for pectus excavatum: a prospective study. Pediatr Surg Int. 2008;24(6):659–66.
13. Bouchard S, Hong AR, Gilchrist BF, Kuenzler KA. Catastrophic cardiac injuries encountered during the minimally invasive repair of pectus excavatum. Semin Pediatr Surg. 2009;18(2):66–72.
14. Vegunta RK, Pacheco PE, Wallace LJ, Pearl RH. Complications associated with the Nuss procedure: continued evolution of the learning curve. Am J Surg. 2008;195(3):313–7.
15. Adam LA, Lawrence JL, Meehan JJ. Erosion of the Nuss bar into the internal mammary artery 4 months after minimally invasive repair of pectus excavatum. J Pediatr Surg. 2008;43(2):394–7.
16. Barsness K, Bruny J, Janik JS, Partrick DA. Delayed near-fatal hemorrhage after Nuss bar displacement. J Pediatr Surg. 2005;40(11):e5–6.
17. Nath DS, Wells WJ, Reemtsen BL. Mechanical occlusion of the inferior vena cava: an unusual complication after repair of pectus excavatum using the Nuss procedure. Ann Thorac Surg. 2008;85(5):1796–8.
18. Ballouhey Q, Léobon B, Trinchéro JF, Baunin C, Galinier P, de Gauzy JS. Mechanical occlusion of the inferior vena cava: an early complication after repair of pectus excavatum using the Nuss procedure. J Pediatr Surg. 2012;47(12):e1–3.
19. Kelly RE, et al. Twenty-one years of experience with minimally invasive repair of pectus excavatum by the Nuss procedure in 1215 patients. Ann Surg. 2010;252(6):1072–81.
20. Nuss D, Obermeyer RJ, Kelly RE. Nuss bar procedure: past, present and future. Ann Cardiothorac Surg. 2016;5(5):422–33.
21. Kelly RE, et al. Multicenter study of pectus excavatum, final report: complications, static/exercise pulmonary function, and anatomic outcomes. J Am Coll Surg. 2013;217(6):1080–9.
22. Morimoto K, Imai K, Yamada A, Fujimoto T, Matsumoto H, Niizuma K. Migration of a pectus bar into the ribs. J Plast Reconstr Aesthet Surg. 2008;61(2):225–7.
23. Raff GW, Wong MS. Sternal plating to correct an unusual complication of the Nuss procedure: erosion of a pectus bar through the sternum. Ann Thorac Surg. 2008;85(3):1100–1.
24. Dalrymple-Hay MJ, Calver A, Lea RE, Monro JL. Migration of pectus excavatum correction bar into the left ventricle. Eur J Cardiothorac Surg. 1997;12(3):507–9.
25. Hoel TN, Rein KA, Svennevig JL. A life-threatening complication of the Nuss-procedure for pectus excavatum. Ann Thorac Surg. 2006;81(1):370–2.
26. Nagasao T, et al. Thoracic outlet syndrome after the Nuss procedure for pectus excavatum: is it a rare complication? J Plast Reconstr Aesthet Surg. 2017;70(10):1433–9.
27. Fox ME, Bensard DD, Brent Roaten J, Hendrickson RJ. Positioning for the Nuss procedure: avoiding brachial plexus injury. Pediatr Anesth. 2005;15(12):1067–71.
28. Peterson RJ, Young JW, Godwin JD, Sabiston JD, Jones RH. Noninvasive assessment of exercise cardiac function before and after pectus excavatum repair. J Thorac Cardiovasc Surg. 1985;90(2):251–60.

29. Shin S, Goretsky MJ, Kelly RE, Gustin T, Nuss D. Infectious complications after the Nuss repair in a series of 863 patients. J Pediatr Surg. 2007;42(1):87–92.
30. Kelly RE, et al. Prospective multicenter study of surgical correction of pectus excavatum: design, perioperative complications, pain, and baseline pulmonary function facilitated by internet-based data collection. J Am Coll Surg. 2007;205(2):205–16.
31. Weber PG, Huemmer HP, Reingruber B. Forces to be overcome in correction of pectus excavatum. J Thorac Cardiovasc Surg. 2006;132(6):1369–73.
32. Chavoin J-P, et al. Correction of pectus excavatum by custom-made silicone implants: contribution of computer-aided design reconstruction. A 20-year experience and 401 cases. Plast Reconstr Surg. 2016;137(5):860e.

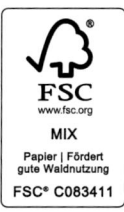

Zeitfracht Medien GmbH
Ferdinand-Jühlke-Straße 7
99095 Erfurt, Deutschland
produktsicherheit@kolibri360.de